Introduction to Gynaecological Endoscopy

Introduction to Gynaecological Endoscopy

Edited by

Adrian M. Lower MRCOG

Consultant Gynaecologist
St Bartholomew's Hospital, London

Christopher J.G. Sutton FRCOG

Director of Minimal Access Therapy Training Unit and
Consultant Gynaecologist
Royal Surrey County Hospital, Guildford
and Chelsea and Westminster Hospital, London

J. Gedis Grudzinskas MD FRCOG

Professor, Department of Obstetrics and Gynaecology
The Royal London Hospital, London, UK

I S I S
MEDICAL
MEDIA

Oxford

© 1996 Isis Medical Media Ltd
58 St Aldates
Oxford OX1 1ST, UK

First published 1996

British Library Cataloguing in Publication Data
A catalogue record for this title is available from the British Library

ISBN   1 899066 28 4

Lower A. (Adrian)
Introduction to Gynaecological Endoscopy/
Adrian Lower, Christopher Sutton, Gedis Grudzinskas

Always refer to the manufacturer's Prescribing Information before prescribing drugs cited in this book

Typeset by
Creative Associates, Oxford, UK

Colour Origination by
Reed Reprographics, Ipswich, UK

Printed by
Dah Hua Printing Press Co., Hong Kong

Distributed by
Times Mirror International Publishers
Customer Service Centre, Unit 1, 3 Sheldon Way,
Larkfield, Aylesford, Kent ME20 6SF, UK

Contents

Contents

Contributors

Salim Bassil MD
Infertility Research Unit, Department of Gynaecology, Catholic University of Louvain, Cliniques Universitaires St Luc, Avenue Hippocrate, 10, B-1200 Brussels, Belgium

Kay F. Donaldson MRCOG
Career Registrar, Southern General Hospital, Govan Road, Glasgow G51 5TF, UK

Jacques G. Donnez MD PhD
Professor and Chairman, Infertility Research Unit, Department of Gynaecology, Catholic University of Louvain, Cliniques Universitaires St Luc, Avenue Hippocrate 10, B-1200 Brussels, Belgium

Simon P. Ewen MB ChB MRCOG
Senior Registrar, Department of Obstetrics and Gynaecology, St Peters Hospital, Guildford Road, Chertsey, Surrey KT16 0PZ, UK

Ray Garry MD FRCOG
Consultant Gynaecologist and Medical Director, The WEL Foundation, South Cleveland Hospital, Marton Road, Middlesbrough, Cleveland TS4 3BW, UK

J. Gedis Grudzinskas MD FRCOG
Professor, Joint Academic Unit of Obstetrics, Gynaecology and Reproductive Physiology, The Royal London Hospital, Whitechapel Road, London E1 1BB, UK

Steven G. Harding MRCOG
Senior Registrar, Fazakerley Hospital, Longmoor Lane, Liverpool L9 7AL, UK

Robert J.S. Hawthorn MD MRCOG
Consultant Gynaecologist, Southern General Hospital, Govan Road, Glasgow G51 5TF, UK

Olav Istre MD PhD
Consultant, The Central Hospital of Hedemark County, N-2300 Hamar, Norway

Adrian M. Lower B Med Sc BM BS MRCOG
Consultant Gynaecologist, St Bartholomew's Hospital, West Smithfield, London EC1, UK

D. Lyndsey McMillan
Whipp's Cross Hospital, Whipp's Cross Road, Leytonstone, London E11 1NR, UK

Michèle Nisolle MD
Infertility Research Unit, Department of Gynaecology, Catholic University of Louvain, Cliniques Universitaires St Luc, Avenue Hippocrate 10, B-1200 Brussels, Belgium

Contributors

Jeffrey H. Phipps BSc MD MRCOG

Unit Director, Consultant Gynaecologist and Medical Bio-Engineer, George Eliot Centre for Minimal Access Gynaecological Surgery, College Street, Nuneaton, Warwickshire, CV10 7DJ, UK

Roland Polet MD

Infertility Research Unit, Department of Gynaecology, Catholic University of Louvain, Cliniques Universitaires St Luc, Avenue Hippocrate 10, B-1200 Brussels, Belgium

Mireille Smets MD

Infertility Research Unit, Department of Gynaecology, Catholic University of Louvain, Cliniques Universitaires St Luc, Avenue Hippocrate 10, B-1200 Brussels, Belgium

Anthony R.B. Smith BSc MD FRCOG

Consultant Gynaecologist, St Mary's Hospital, Whitworth Park, Manchester M13 OJH, UK

Christopher J.G. Sutton FRCOG

Consultant Gynaecologist, Chelsea and Westminster Hospital, Fulham Road, Chelsea, London SW10 9NH, UK

Geoffrey H. Trew MB BS MRCOG

Consultant in Reproductive Medicine, Institute of Obstetrics and Gynaecology, Hammersmith Hospital, Du Cane Road, London W12 OHS, UK

Foreword

With the explosive development of endoscopic surgery, particularly in gynaecology, it is appropriate that a new textbook should be devoted to this rapidly developing subject. The authors are a splendid mix of youthful enthusiasm combined with the experience of some of the foremost exponents of minimal access surgery in the world. The authors represent contemporary opinion from both busy district hospitals and major university teaching centres. The majority of the authors are British, but there are important contributions from the internationally famous group of endoscopic surgeons from Louvain, Belgium and a contribution on hysteroscopic complications from Norway. As the title implies, this is an introduction to gynaecological endoscopic surgery with great emphasis on training standards and safety.

The Royal College of Obstetricians and Gynaecologists and the British Society for Gynaecological Endoscopy have had a major influence in introducing agreed standards for training for young surgeons and implementing a validation mechanism supervised by the Royal College. These recent advances represent a significant contribution to patient safety by ensuring inexperienced surgeons operate with adequate supervision. The strong emphasis in the book on training, equipment and instruments, should help to persuade hospitals to invest in purchasing 'state–of–the–art' equipment for the operating theatre, with financial encouragement to surgeons at all levels to attend national and international training courses and conferences. No operating theatre can function efficiently without adequately trained scrub nurses to look after the instruments, and this aspect is emphasized. Few surgeons understand the mechanism of electrosurgery and why diathermy injuries to patients occur. This volume seeks to educate the beginner in the basic principles of electrical energy.

Surgical lasers are expensive, but add greatly to the surgeon's versatility and in institutions where large numbers of patients are treated, the unit cost of treatment falls dramatically and operations become cost effective.

After the introductory chapters, individual operations are discussed, described and criticized in great detail by recognised leaders in the profession renowned for the clarity of their presentation as well as their clinical expertise. The chapters are deliberately didactic as appropriate for a teaching manual for embryonic minimal access surgeons. The operations range from basic laparoscopic surgery, such as tubal sterilization (which is often performed extremely badly and is the source of much litigation) to the most advanced laparoscopic procedures and are profusely illustrated with line drawings and photographs. Both the indications and contra-indications to surgery are emphasized and every step of each operation is minutely described together with common technical difficulties and how to solve them. An interesting and novel feature are the panels containing key points and safety advice which are especially helpful.

Many of the common gynaecological operations now performed by laparotomy, can be safely performed through the operating laparoscope, the limits to surgery are probably set by individual training and experience rather than technical difficulty. The undoubted benefits of early discharge from hospital and a rapid return to work should not be unavailable because of lack of experience. Nevertheless, it is still a fundamental necessity that junior doctors must be trained in classical surgery before embarking on the fascinating sub–specialty of minimal access surgery. The beginner must be able to recognize the limits of this technical expertise and be prepared to convert laparoscopic surgery to classical laparotomy if insuperable technical difficulties supervene. With increasing experience, conversion to laparotomy will occur less frequently.

Foreword

This new volume will undoubtedly be a major contribution to the sub–specialty, and will encourage doctors training to understand the scope of laparoscopic surgery and above all, contribute to the evaluation and audit of laparoscopic and hysteroscopic operations. This book should be in all postgraduate libraries and be read by both junior doctors and their senior colleagues. Only by maintaining the highest technical and critical standards will the sub–specialty of minimal access surgery continue its inexorable advance, be accepted by hospital managers , and expected by our patients.

B. Victor Lewis
MD FRCS FRCOG
Past President
British Society for Gynaecological Endoscopy

Preface

The concept of this book was realised following a series of successful advanced gynaecological endoscopy courses during 1994 and 1995. The Editors are grateful to the members of faculty and delegates attending these courses for their encouragement and support of this book.

The book reached the stage of publication in a relatively short period of time thanks to the enthusiasm and diligence of the publishers and contributors. The Editors would also like to express their sincere thanks and appreciation of their wives and families for their continuing acceptance of our passion for surgery and publication.

We have received many helpful comments and letters of advice from our students and from teachers all over the world.

We hope that this book finds favour internationally and helps to promote the practice of safe endoscopic gynaecological surgery.

Adrian M. Lower
Christopher J.G. Sutton
J. Gedis Grudzinskas

Chapter 1
Introduction
A.M. Lower, C.J.G. Sutton and J.G. Grudzinskas

A surgical revolution

Who should read this book

How to use this book

A surgical revolution

The 1970s and 1980s witnessed a revolution in surgical technique, not only in gynaecology but in several other branches of surgery. Early attempts at endoscopy were hampered by poor optical systems and the need to introduce light in some way to illuminate the internal cavities. The invention of the rod lens system by Professor H. Hopkins FRS at the University of Reading, coupled with his other invention of fibre optic cables to transport the light from a source outside the body, was largely responsible for the view we have today on our video monitors, which enables us to inspect the inside of the uterus or the peritoneal cavity with extraordinary clarity. We owe him an enormous debt for the high-quality optics that we enjoy in endoscopy today. Most of the pioneering innovations in endoscopic surgery came from such people as Raoul Palmer of Paris and Hans Frangenheim of Konstanz, who were the forefathers of modern laparoscopic surgery but largely confined their techniques to female sterilization and simple aspiration of ovarian cysts. Patrick Steptoe learned from them, and by publishing his book[1] on laparoscopic surgery in the 1950s led to the wide dissemination of knowledge about laparoscopy in the English-speaking countries. Even then, the procedure was largely used for diagnosis and simple operations like uterine ventrosuspension and early techniques of ovum collection, which led to the birth of the first test-tube baby, Louise Brown, in 1978.

It is estimated that about 80% of gynaecological operations that required laparotomy can now be performed by laparoscopic surgery. The main impetus for this came from Kurt Semm and his team at the University of Kiel in Northern Germany and Professor Maurice Bruhat and Hubert Manhes from the Auvergne in France. Laser laparoscopy was first performed by a Bruhat team[2] in 1979, but then largely neglected in favour of electrosurgical techniques. Laparoscopic laser surgery was first reported in North America by Jim Daniell from Nashville, Tennessee. It was introduced into the UK by Chris Sutton from Guildford, Surrey, and popularized in Europe by Jacques Donnez from Brussels.

When we first started using the carbon dioxide laser through the laparoscope in October 1982, our first concern was to ensure that the technique was absolutely safe when used correctly. Our greatest fear was a methane explosion from inadvertent perforation of the bowel with the laser beam, and we constructed a worst-case scenario: employing a freshly removed section of the colon and working in an atmosphere firstly of air and later of carbon dioxide, we deliberately perforated the specimen but were unable to induce a methane explosion. We knew, from work with the carbon dioxide laser on the cervix, that the laser crater healed with virtually no fibrosis or scarring, which resulted in healing without any anatomical distortion, and we had evidence from animal work conducted by Bellina in New Orleans that the rabbit peritoneum healed in a similar way – indeed, it was difficult to detect where the laser surgery had taken place. We also knew that the main disadvantage of the laser was its poor haemostatic capabilities when vessels larger than capillaries were transected, and we were careful to have additional haemostatic equipment available. (In those days the safest was Semm's endocoagulator, which Semm had developed to coagulate tissue to avoid the dangers associated with the electrosurgical equipment that was available at that time.)

From these tentative early surgical endeavours the adoption of endoscopic techniques has spread rapidly.

Who should read this book

This book is designed to be a practical guide for trainees in gynaecological surgery and more senior gynaecologists who wish to develop new skills in endoscopic surgery. It covers the principal learning points required for progress through routine diagnostic videolaparoscopy to advanced operative procedures.

The approach is predominantly visual and practical, with guidance on selected references for further reading.

How to use this book

This book provides sound advice and background to the procedures employed. The early chapters review the place of training and the equipment available. Noted experts then address particular procedures.

After studying the basic information included in these chapters, trainees should ensure that they are thoroughly familiar with the equipment available in their own hospitals. This familiarity must be achieved by performing all diagnostic procedures with the video equipment, and gradually progressing to minor operative procedures such as tubal ligation. Procedures should initially be performed under direct supervision; later, supervision can be maintained by review of video recordings of operative procedures. Once familiarity has been obtained with minor procedures, trainees will progress to performing under supervision the simpler stages of more advanced procedures, e.g. treatment of the posterior wall of the uterus in transcervical resection of the endometrium, or the stapling of the upper pedicles at laparoscopic hysterectomy. Once the trainer is satisfied with the competence of trainees in these procedures, trainees will progress to performing complete procedures under direct supervision and later under indirect supervision by review of video recordings. This training programme is summarized overleaf.

Training programme

1. Acquire sound theoretical knowledge
2. Become thoroughly familiar with equipment through diagnostic procedures
3. Assist and observe operative procedures
4. Perform simple procedures under direct supervision
5. Perform simpler stages of advanced procedures under supervision
6. Perform complete procedures under direct supervision
7. Operate under indirect supervison
8. Audit of operations

Chapter 2 discusses in more detail the RCOG guidelines on training in endoscopic surgery and expands on the necessity to attend recognized training courses.

Our aim is to communicate the state of art in endoscopic surgery so that readers will feel confident to join the growing ranks of surgeons who are embracing this new and challenging technique.

References

1. Steptoe P C (1967) Laparoscopy and gynaecology. Livingstone, London.
2. Bruhat M, Mages C, Manhes H (1979) Use of CO_2 laser via laparoscopy. In: Kaplan I (ed.) Laser surgery III. *Proceedings of the third congress of the International Society for Laser Surgery.* Jerusalem Press, Tel Aviv, pp. 275–81.

Chapter 2

Structured Training in Endoscopic Surgery

C.J.G. Sutton and A.M. Lower

Introduction

This chapter looks at the background behind the requirement to develop structured training in gynaecological endoscopy. It reviews the place and development of the MATTU centres, and the published recommendations of the RCOG Working Party on Training in Gynaecological Endoscopic Surgery and their implementation.

Background

The early pioneers in endoscopic surgery were largely self-taught; however, an analysis of their work shows that it was done with considerable caution, in a logical progressive manner and accompanied by careful audit. As their skills developed, and they made progress from relatively simple procedures to ones of increasing complexity, they inevitably encountered some of the advanced procedures with which they were unfamiliar. The majority of surgeons would visit a colleague who had developed expertise with the procedure and observe him or her at work, and encourage an expert in that particular technique to visit their institution so that they might acquire the necessary instruction before attempting to perform the technique themselves.

With the rapid evolution of endoscopic surgery and its wider dissemination into different hospitals it is regrettable that the same careful progression from simple to difficult cases has not always occurred. Some surgeons have merely attended a course or watched a few videos and have then embarked on complicated procedures without any fundamental training; often the staff in the operating theatre are unfamiliar with the equipment and the problems that can arise very rapidly during endoscopic surgery. It was inevitable that accidents should occur, some of them serious or even fatal. To avoid this, more formalized training is being developed both at the Royal College of Surgeons (RCS) and the Royal College of Obstetricians and Gynaecologists (RCOG). A number of training institutions have also emerged.

Minimal Access Therapy Training Unit (MATTU)

In 1992 the Department of Health in conjunction with the Wolfson Foundation provided substantial funds with the aim of improving training in minimal access surgery in an attempt to reduce the growing number of surgical accidents. Bids were invited from interested parties to establish national training centres in minimally invasive surgery funded by this joint initiative. Some 120 hospitals put in bids, and the shortlisted units had to present themselves to a panel at the Department of Health in Leeds on 7 June 1993. The panel chose to support three major minimal access therapy training units (MATTUs), the main one to be based at the Royal College of Surgeons, incorporating the Raven Department of Education and linked to clinical centres at the Royal London Hospital and the Royal Surrey County Hospital in Guildford. A further MATTU was sited at the United Leeds Teaching Hospitals, with clinical help in gynaecology from Ray Garry and his team from the South Cleveland Hospital in Middlesborough. A further centre under the general direction of Professor Alfred Cuschieri was to be based in Dundee, with assistance in gynaecology from endoscopic surgeons in Perth, Glasgow and Edinburgh.

The funding has enabled these units to be equipped with advanced, state-of-the-art teaching and simulation facilities (Figure 2.1), including interactive computer-assisted learning workstations, simulators incorporating dual video monitors and advanced endoscopic cameras, and sophisticated audiovisual systems that allow speakers to move between overhead projectors, slide projectors and video by touch screen control. In addition to standard slide projection they can use computer-generated slides, videotape, a flat bed visualizer, CD ROM and laser disks of still images. The RCS MATTU is connected by live audiovisual links to the operating theatres of its major clinical partners, the Royal London Hospital and the Royal Surrey County Hospital.

The RCS MATTU was officially opened in 1995. Courses are run in surgical skills on the simulators in the MATTU, and separate courses are run at the Royal Surrey County Hospital and the Royal London Hospital. The RCS has also started a series of Training the Trainers courses to improve the quality of training and ensure uniformity in

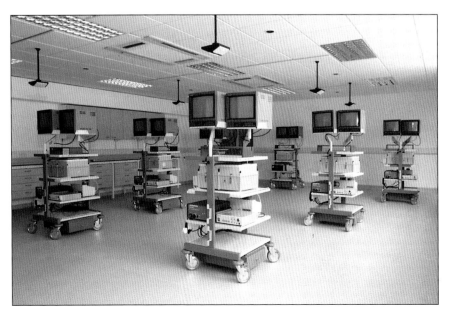

Figure 2.1 *A state-of-the-art teaching and simulation facility (courtesy of Mr Frank Sambrook, RCS).*

approach. These courses, under the direction of Professor Duncan Morris, Professor of Education at Brunel University, and Mr Rodney Peyton from Northern Ireland, who has taught the trainers on the highly successful Advanced Trauma and Life Support Training Scheme run by the RCS, teach experienced surgeons very valuable lessons in how to teach essentially practical skills. This is something which most of us would agree many of our own teachers sadly lacked, despite being gifted and inspiring surgeons.

RCOG guidelines

In June 1994 the RCOG published the report of the Working Party on Training in Gynaecological Endoscopic Surgery, which was under the Chairmanship of Professor Robert Shaw from Cardiff. The full report can be obtained from the RCOG Book Shop at a price of £7, but has been circulated free to fellows and members of the College.

The RCOG recognized that operative endoscopy represents a rapidly increasing component of gynaecological surgery, and the Education Board, under the Chairmanship of Dr Naren Patel, realized that education in this type of surgery must be addressed rapidly as a result of surgical complications which have arisen related to these new procedures. Section 1 of the Working Party Report states that 'Surgeons who begin to perform these new techniques must acquire new equipment but a far greater need is to appreciate the training in hand and eye coordination required for endoscopic surgical procedures'. With these problems in mind, it was felt that a framework was needed for training in order to provide the maximum support to clinicians while they endeavour to gain these new skills and until the new techniques have become widespread and accessible to most trainees who could be taught them as a routine component in their structured training programmes.

The RCOG agreed to recognize the MATTUs and that a further Working Party should be set up to agree on the content for recognized courses. It was further agreed that no commercially run courses would be accepted unless they met the guidelines set by the Minimal Access Surgery Training Subcommittee.

Stratification of laparoscopic and hysteroscopic procedures by levels of training

The main achievement of the Working Party was to look at the various procedures that were being performed endoscopically and to devise levels of increasing difficulty in both laparoscopic and hysteroscopic surgery. The levels identified are shown below:

Laparoscopic procedures

Level 1: Diagnostic laparoscopy

Level 2: Minor laparoscopic procedures
- Laparoscopic sterilization
- Needle aspiration of simple cysts
- Ovarian biopsy
- Minor adhesiolysis (not involving bowel)
- Diathermy for endometriosis – revised American Fertility Society stage I
- Diathermy for polycystic ovaries
- Linear salpingostomy and/or salpingectomy for ectopic pregnancy

Level 3: More extensive procedures requiring additional training
- Laser treatment for polycystic ovaries
- Laser treatment or diathermy for endometriosis – revised American Fertility Society stages II and III
- Laparoscopic uterosacral nerve ablation
- Salpingostomy for infertility
- Salpingo-oophorectomy
- Adhesiolysis for moderate bowel adhesions
- Laparoscopic ovarian cystectomy
- Laparoscopic or laser management of endometrioma
- Laparoscopically assisted vaginal hysterectomy
- Laparoscopic subtotal hysterectomy (without significant associated pathology)

Level 4: Extensive endoscopic procedures requiring subspecialist or advanced/tertiary level endoscopic skills
- Laparoscopic hysterectomy with associated pathology
- Total hysterectomy
- Myomectomy
- Laparoscopic surgery for revised American Fertility Society stage III and IV endometriosis
- Pelvic lymphadenectomy
- Pelvic side-wall or ureteric dissection
- Presacral neurectomy
- Dissection of an obliterated pouch of Douglas
- Laparoscopic incontinence procedures
- Laparoscopic suspension procedures

In the original RCOG Working Party Report ventrosuspension was included in the laparoscopy group, but this has now been withdrawn as it is a relatively uncommon procedure and many trainees would not have an opportunity to receive the necessary training.

Hysteroscopic procedures

Level 1: Simple procedures
- Diagnostic hysteroscopy plus target biopsy
- Removal of simple polyps
- Removal of intrauterine contraceptive devices

Level 2: Minor operative procedures
- Proximal fallopian tube cannulation
- Minor Asherman's syndrome
- Removal of pedunculated fibroids or large polyps

Level 3: More complex operative procedures requiring additional training
- Division or resection of uterine septa
- Endoscopic surgery for major Asherman's syndrome
- Endometrial resection or ablation
- Resection of submucous leiomyoma
- Repeat endometrial resection or ablation

It is expected that all MRCOG trainees should become competent in level 1 and 2 laparoscopic procedures and level 1 hysteroscopic procedures by the end of their basic training. Progress beyond these levels will require further teaching.

There has been some controversy about the inclusion of laparoscopic surgery for the treatment of unruptured ectopic pregnancies on the basis that some people from overseas might not have access to this equipment in their own countries and that many units in the UK are still not performing laparoscopic surgery for unruptured ectopic pregnancies. Nevertheless, the Committee was adamant that this level of competence should be required during the training of a registrar, because the laparoscopic treatment of unruptured tubal pregnancy is one of the few procedures that has been shown to be the gold standard of treatment by properly designed prospective randomized clinical studies. It was felt, therefore, that this would provide an impetus for units that are deficient in these skills at the moment to enable their administrations to provide adequate equipment and for the consultants at these institutions to get the necessary training to be able to teach their juniors to a satisfactory standard for the MRCOG examination.

Implementation of the RCOG Working Party recommendations

This Committee, again under the Chairmanship of Professor Robert Shaw, and with representatives from the British Society of Gynaecological Endoscopy and the established MATTUs, and other surgeons and educators, is at present working out how this training is to be implemented. The Working Party has not finished its work and has not yet reported to either Council or the Education Committee of the RCOG but already certain proposals seem likely.

Training centres

A number of designated training centres will be recognized by the RCOG. It is hoped that the course content of the MATTUs will be standardized and certain skills will be measured at the beginning and end of each course. Many of the skills tests are easily reproducible and can be measured on a scoring system; only if trainees acquire the necessary skills will they be awarded a certificate and allowed to move on to a higher level. Attendance at these courses will not necessarily result in obtaining a certificate, and courses run by other centres will be recognized by the RCOG only if they can be shown to achieve the same standards and if the centres allow themselves to be inspected by designated RCOG representatives.

Proposed training

Levels 1 and 2

The Committee is almost certain to decide that all trainee specialists in obstetrics and gynaecology must attend a recognized fundamental course incorporating the basic skills required for both laparoscopy and hysteroscopy. These courses should be attended at an early stage in the registrar's training, and a certificate of attendance at such a recognized course would be required for final membership of the RCOG. To proceed to higher training in endoscopic surgery, a certificate of competence will be required in hand–eye coordination skills and a knowledge of the technical equipment used in this type of surgery.

The skills required for levels 1 and 2 will be assessed at the place of work by MRCOG trainers as an integral part of the formative and summative assessment for the membership examination. It will be a normal part of structured training. It is recognized that it is not possible to develop the hand–eye coordination necessary to work from a video screen overnight and, arguably, the single most important factor in helping to train for operative endoscopy is that *all* diagnostic procedures should be performed using the video monitor. Trainees will thus become entirely familiar with the two-dimensional environment and progress more quickly in all their operative work.

Levels 3 and 4

Gynaecologists wishing to proceed to these levels should already have obtained a certificate of competence at levels 1 and 2, and would be expected to attend an RCOG-recognized advanced course. Provided they demonstrate the attainment of an adequate level of skill on completion of such a course, they would be given a certificate of attendance. Trainees would be expected to obtain expert supervision from a preceptor recognized by the RCOG, firstly in assisting with these operations and then in performing them under supervision on a one-to-one basis. The trainee would have to register with the RCOG accordingly and undergo a period of intensive training, which would include critical analysis of video recordings, technical knowledge of the equipment and the energy sources used and a thorough knowledge of the literature concerning these operations. Following satisfactory reports the RCOG will probably issue a certificate of competence, which could be required by hospitals both in the National Health Service and in the private sector before accrediting the surgeon to perform procedures at this level. This certificate of competence would also be helpful in the event of a complication occurring and would provide evidence of satisfactory training. From the time of the acquisition of the certificate the individual concerned would be enrolled in the appropriate Continuing Medical Education (CME) programme on a 5 yearly basis, assuming that they wished to have these skills re-certified.

Subspecialty training

Many of the procedures at level 4 are likely to be performed only by subspecialists or in tertiary referral centres for endoscopic surgery: the urogynaecologist will concentrate on laparoscopic incontinence procedures and laparoscopic pelvic floor repairs and is unlikely to need the skills of pelvic lymphadenectomy and pelvic sidewall dissection, which are the provenance of the gynaecological oncologist.

Conclusion

The implementation of these recommendations is going to be a major task in the initial phases but, once endoscopic surgery becomes part of the normal training schedule for registrars, endoscopic surgery will become part of the apprenticeship system in much the same way as training in abdominal or vaginal hysterectomy is at present.

At present, the British Society of Gynaecological Endoscopy and the RCOG Working Party are drawing up a list of suitable trainers. It is evident that there are many who can give audited proof of their competence in endoscopic surgery; they will be designated 'grandparents' and will not have to attend courses for which they have already adequately demonstrated their skills. It is hoped, however, that they will take part in a Training the Trainers course and will be prepared to help with the surgical skills laboratories at the basic training courses and to take on trainees for proctoring or preceptorships.

Probably the greatest difficulty will be with some consultants who feel that they are too close to retirement to justify embarking on this very extensive training programme, and this is a particular problem with consultants who might be carrying out one endoscopic procedure, such as endometrial ablation, but very little in the way of laparoscopic surgery apart from very simple procedures. Nevertheless, it is recommended that consultants who wish to be recognized as experienced hysteroscopists and laparoscopists should undertake the same training programme as that recommended for trainees. They would need to be registered with the Minimum Access Surgery Training Subcommittee and have their training programme recognized, and following the completion of this programme they would be duly certified.

It must be realized that this kind of surgery is not for everyone: some consultants may choose not to practise minimal access surgery, and they should not be coerced into doing so, but equally they should not try to practise this kind of surgery without evidence of satisfactory training. It must also be realized that some people are innately unable to achieve the necessary eye–hand coordination to perform these techniques, using a video monitor, safely. Professor Alfred Cuschieri from Dundee estimates that this number may be as high as 13%. These colleagues should be informed of this and gently steered into the numerous other areas of interest that exist within our specialty. The concept of aptitude testing for surgeons is difficult for many to accept; however, the precedent has been set in other professions where a high degree of skill and coordination is required – airline pilots and even car drivers must have a licence. It is better for the profession to accept self-regulation and assessment than to have it imposed by outside agencies.

Finally, surgeons must also be willing to submit their work to audit and, where an unacceptable rate of complications is found, be prepared to amend their practice or face retraining.

Summary

Rapid advances in endoscopic surgical techniques and their wider applicability to gynaecological diseases no longer permit the luxury of a surgeon to be self-taught in often complex procedures. The Department of Health in the UK have taken the initiative to develop a number of training centres to ensure that these necessary skills are acquired by surgeons under guidance and in a structured manner. The RCOG has recommended that there is a stratification of laparoscopic and hysteroscopic procedures by levels of training to ensure the acquisition of these skills is accessible to gynaecologists at all stages of their career development with particular reference in the doctor-in-training. It is intended that all RCOG trainees will reach levels of expertise, I and II, in diagnostic and minor laparoscopic procedures. The more complex procedures listed in levels III and IV will be acquired at a peri– or post–consultant level of career advancement, experience for the most complex procedures in subspecialist areas being acquired by subspecialists in reproductive medicine, oncology and uro-gynaecology.

Chapter 3
Laboratory Training
A.M. Lower

Introduction

This chapter explores the requirement to use models to assist in the development of hand–eye coordination for endoscopic surgery. The discussion includes: the use of simple models to improve hand–eye coordination; the use of more sophisticated latex models, which more faithfully reproduce normal anatomy; and the use of animal models, either animals under terminal anaesthesia or fresh cadaver specimens.

The final part of this chapter includes a series of structured exercises using small bowel and ovary to simulate gynaecological tissue.

Hand–eye coordination

Inanimate models serve a useful purpose in helping to develop hand–eye coordination and the ability to work from the video screen. Such models also serve to improve the surgeon's familiarity with the video equipment, including the light source, camera and monitor. It is essential that the surgeon has a thorough understanding of the operation of this equipment and how it should be connected together, in addition to the ability to perform basic fault-finding tests if a picture cannot be obtained. The following is a list of exercises that have been used to good effect for this important aspect of training.

Exercises

Pegboards and rubber bands

In this model, a number of pins or nails are placed in a wooden board Rubber bands can be placed from pin to pin and moved from one pin to another. This offers the surgeon exercise in appreciating the depth of field and operating in a three-dimensional environment using only a two-dimensional video screen for cues. Cutting and clipping the rubber bands can also be practised using scissors or clips as appropriate.

Placing matches in a matchbox

This simple idea has been used on our courses to test the surgeon's ability to work in three dimensions. A matchbox is placed in the

Key point

The ability to work from the video screen is essential.

Bodyform cabinet, initially closed. The trainee surgeon is then required to open the matchbox and remove the matches, placing them on the surface adjacent to the box and then replacing them in the box. This tests the ability to move and manipulate irregularly shaped objects within the three-dimensional environment. We have held competitions in which trainees are timed completing this task, which has generated an air of friendly rivalry and helped to develop relationships at the beginning of courses.

Dried peas

Dried peas are an interesting model because their shape and texture make them difficult to grasp with forceps. These can be placed into a gallipot and then removed again. This provides practice in the appreciation of depth and awareness of three-dimensional control using the two-dimensional video screen.

Grapes

Grapes form a useful model, although they tend to contaminate the instruments more than the examples used above. Peeling a grape without detaching it from the stalk is a fairly demanding test of the trainee surgeon's ability to work from the video screen and to grasp fragile structures such as the ovary without causing trauma.

Foam trees

Foam trees are available from commercial sources and provide a good model on which to practise stapling and clipping. The foam models are not particularly life-like, but they do serve to simulate tissue in an inexpensive and readily obtainable fashion. They can also be used for practising suturing and cutting.

Latex models

Once surgeons have developed familiarity with models of the type listed above, their ability to perform surgical procedures can be tested using latex models that faithfully reproduce the anatomy of the female pelvis. These are commercially available from Limbs & Things, Bristol, UK. Figure 3.1 shows the BodyForm cabinet, which can be sealed to allow creation of a pneumoperitoneum. This can be used to train in the correct technique for trocar insertion (Figure 3.2). Life-like latex models of the pelvic organs can be placed in the BodyForm cabinet, correctly positioned within a model of the bony pelvis (Figure 3.3).

Models can be used to simulate different dissections to train surgeons in various procedures. Figure 3.4 shows a model of the bladder and vagina, which are pegged to maintain their position. Material is held in place over the pubic crest so that the placing of sutures can be practised.

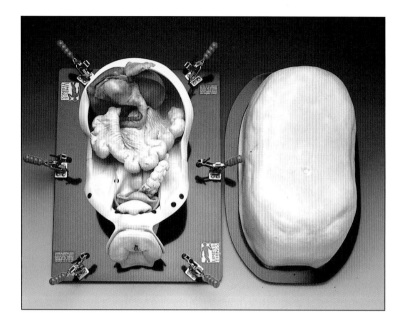

Figure 3.1 *BodyForm cabinet (courtesy of Limbs & Things, Bristol, UK).*

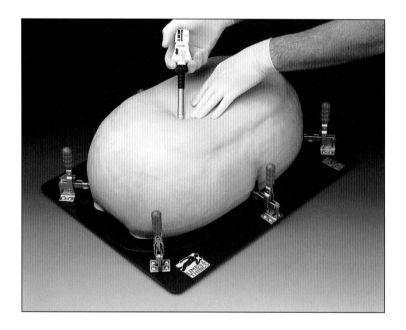

Figure 3.2 *Trocar insertion using the BodyForm cabinet (courtesy of Limbs and Things, Bristol, UK).*

However, the models are relatively expensive and, although the key structures are present and the tissue handles somewhat similarly to living tissue, there are a number of limitations. In particular, the tissue does not bleed when haemostasis has not been adequately achieved.

Animate models

At the time of writing, the UK Home Office regulations concerning the use of animals in medical practice specifically prohibit their use for

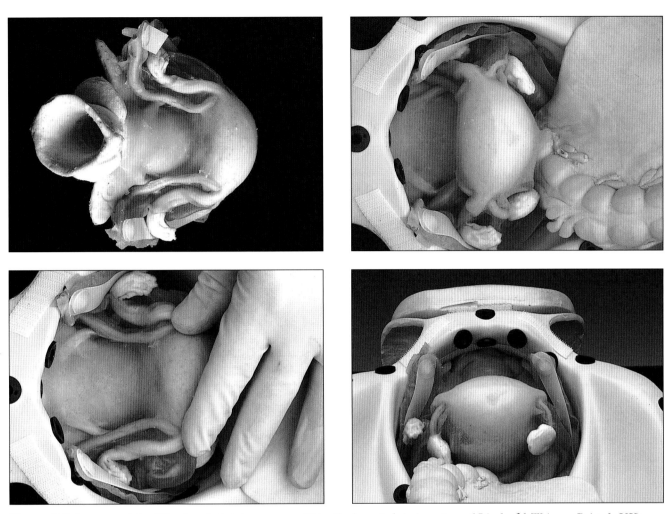

Figure 3.3 *Latex models of the female pelvic organs within the bony pelvis (courtesy of Limbs & Things, Bristol, UK).*

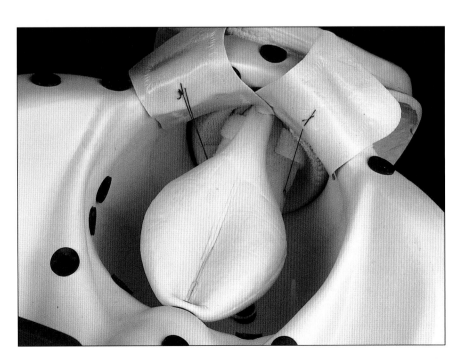

Figure 3.4 *Bladder and vagina assembly for training in colposuspension techniques (courtesy of Limbs & Things, Bristol, UK).*

training purposes, apart from training in microsurgery. They are widely used for training purposes in the USA, and elsewhere in Europe. Generally, the animals are operated on under terminal anaesthesia. A veterinary surgeon is available at all times to ensure adequate levels of analgesia and anaesthesia in the animals. A number of suitable animals have been suggested, including the goat, sheep and pig. The pig is probably the most commonly used model for gynaecological procedures.

The training facilities are equipped to normal operating theatre standard with all the commonly available instrumentation required for endoscopic surgery (Figure 3.5).

This type of model has a number of advantages. The surgeon is able to operate in a familiar operating theatre environment without any of the additional pressures experienced during the course of normal surgery. The tissue has a natural feel and will bleed and behave in exactly the same way as human tissue subjected to electrocautery or laser energy. There are some disadvantages (Table 3.1), of which the moral and ethical aspects of working on animals are perhaps

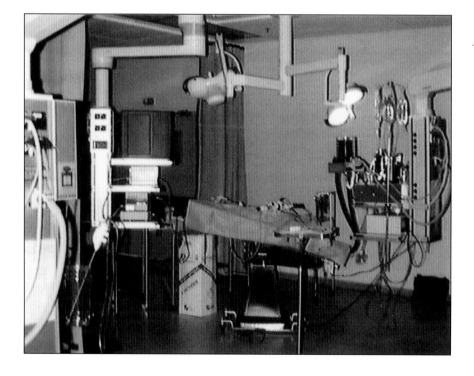

Figure 3.5 *Laboratory training facilities.*

Advantages	Disadvantages
Realistic tissue handling	Illegal in the UK
Practice in the management of complications	Ethical considerations
	Expense
Practice in developmental surgery	Anatomical differences

Table 3.1 *Advantages and disadvantages of animal models*

paramount. Most surgeons undertaking this type of training, and certainly most surgeons running training facilities of this type, believe that the greater good is served by ensuring that surgeons are thoroughly trained in the use of all surgical methods before they attempt such surgery in humans. A detailed examination of the philosophical arguments is beyond the scope of this book. Suffice it to say that, in our experience, surgeons gain immeasurably in confidence after just one operating session of this kind during the course of their training. If you are able to resolve the moral dilemma facing any surgeon making a decision to participate in this form of training, it is to be highly commended.

The other major difficulty in using animal models is the difference in anatomy from humans. To overcome these differences, a number of exercises are described below in which the small bowel of the pig is used to simulate many of the procedures commonly encountered in gynaecological surgery. These exercises take trainee gynaecologists through a series of structured exercises, gaining the maximum benefit from a single operating session of 6–8 hours.

Review of equipment and instrumentation
- Review of peripheral hardware, including video equipment, light source, camera, suction irrigator and carbon dioxide insufflator
- Review of operating instruments, disposable and reusable

Objective: Familiarization with the tools necessary for laparoscopic surgery

Establish pneumoperitoneum
- Use of the Veress needle and alternative insufflation sites
- Manoeuvres to employ when the risk of adhesions is high

Objective: Safe establishment of pneumoperitoneum

Port placement
- Discussion of the best port sites for different procedures
- Familiarization with safety aspects
- Avoidance of blood vessels
- Insertion of trocars under direct vision

Objective: Safe and appropriate insertion of trocars

Identification of porcine anatomy
- Understanding the limitations of the pig model

Tissue-handling exercises
- 'Walking' the bowel
- Use of traumatic and atraumatic forceps

Objective: Safe manipulation of tissue with appropriate instrumentation

Laboratory training

Achieving haemostasis
- Identification and elevation of the mesentery of the small bowel
- Isolation of mesenteric blood vessels
- Use of electrocautery, clips and staples to achieve haemostasis
- Creation of a window in the mesentery using scissors

Objective: Safe and effective establishment of haemostasis
Objective: Safe and effective use of electrocautery
Objective: Precise use of instrumentation

Simulated salpingectomy and appendicectomy
- Use of a linear stapler to transect the bowel after creating a window in the mesentery (a model for the appendix or fallopian tube)
- Application of two Surgitie (Auto Suture, Ascot, UK) or Endoloop (Ethicon, Edinburgh, UK)) ligating loops or a linear stapler to divide the proximal end of the 'tube' to simulate salpingectomy
- Use of a retrieval bag to remove a bowel segment from the peritoneal cavity

Objective: Practice of alternative methods for salpingectomy
Objective: Practice of methods of tissue retrieval

Simulated ectopic pregnancy
- Open section of bowel or uterine horn using electrosurgery, scissors or laser
- Closure using intracorporeal or extracorporeal knots

Objective: Use of different methods to create a salpingostomy
Objective: Observation of different haemostatic properties
Objective: Practice of suturing technique

Oophorectomy
- Use of a linear stapler or electrocautery to remove an ovary
- Use of a retrieval bag to remove an ovary from the peritoneal cavity

Objective: Practice of a method of oophorectomy
Objective: Practice of tissue retrieval avoiding contamination

Drainage of an ovarian cyst
- Use of a Veress needle and suction to drain a bladder

Objective: Simulation of drainage of an ovarian cyst

Simulated laparoscopic hysterectomy
- Application of a linear staple gun to the broad ligament of the uterus

Objective: Simulation of ligation and division of pedicles of the uterus

Colposuspension

- Dissection of the peritoneum anterior to the bladder to open the cave of Retzius using sharp and blunt dissection and electrosurgery where appropriate
- Identification of the bladder neck if possible
- Suture of paravesical tissue or the bladder to the ileopectineal ligament using an extracorporeal knotting technique (the porcine pelvis is much narrower than the human, so suturing the bladder, rather than the paravesical tissue, is a satisfactory model)

Objective: Practice of dissecting skills and appropriate use of electrosurgery for haemostasis

Objective: Insertion of suspensory sutures at laparoscopy

Radical procedures

- Dissection of the peritoneum from the pelvic sidewall and identification of anatomy
- Transection of the ureter and reanastomosis
- Side-to-side bowel anastomosis using a linear stapler and sutures

Objective: Practice of more advanced dissecting skills and surgical procedures

Port closure

- Use Endoclose (Auto Suture, Ascot, UK) or the Rocket J-shaped needle (Rocket, London, UK) to close abdominal incisions

Objective: Practice of sound repair of incisions

Summary

The use of models and laboratory training enables a structured training programme to be followed by all surgeons. There is no risk to the patient, and the surgeon is not faced with the pressure of time that exists in the operating theatre.

Chapter 4

Choosing Equipment for Gynaecological Endoscopy

A.M. Lower

Introduction

This chapter reviews the range of equipment available for laparoscopic surgery. The essential features of each type of instrument are discussed and guidance is provided for those with responsibility for purchasing instruments for endoscopic surgery.

Reusable versus single-use instruments

There is now a large range of instrumentation available. The choice can be daunting for the beginner with limited experience. The first decision that needs to be made is whether to use reusable or single-use instruments. The advantages and disadvantages are summarized in Table 4.1. Most, but not all, instruments are available in reusable and single-use form. Some instruments are more suited to single use than others, particularly cutting and stapling instruments with complicated mechanisms. It is reassuring to know that the risk of instrument failure is low in such cases. In general, single-use instruments are perceived as being more expensive than reusable instruments. However, the cost of cleaning, sterilizing, packing and replacing reusable instruments must be taken into account. Some risk management assessors are recommending the use of single-use instruments to avoid completely the very low risk of cross-infection.

It can also be useful to use single-use instruments at the early stages of one's endoscopic surgical career, deferring expensive capital purchases of instruments until strong preferences have been made and a small number of regularly used instruments have been identified. This is particularly the case at present, because the pace of development of new instruments is fast.

Imaging equipment

The first rule of good surgical practice is to ensure that there is adequate exposure. Endoscopic surgery is no different. The first rule here is to ensure that the image quality is as high as possible. To

Table 4.1 *Advantages and disadvantages of reusable and single-use instruments*

Reusable instruments	Single-use instruments
Probably lower cost per use	High cost
Usually a better engineered feel	No risk of cross-infection
Can be repaired	Guaranteed reliability

Safety point

It is not possible to operate safely unless the image is clear and adequately illuminated.

---

achieve this, it is essential that the camera, monitor, endoscopes, light source and connection cables are of the highest quality and in good condition. Adequate illumination is essential to produce a clear image.

There is some benefit in obtaining this high-cost equipment from the same manufacturer to ensure full compatibility when components are connected, to exploit the technical advantages of the complete system.

Camera

A bewildering range of cameras is now available. The first-generation single-chip cameras lack sensitivity and image quality. The newer three-chip cameras have improved performance, but require higher levels of illumination to function adequately and will not perform optimally if the light connection cables or scopes are showing signs of deterioration.

The resolution of the camera is determined by the number of lines recorded. For most practical purposes the S-VHS standard of 625 lines is adequate. This can be achieved with some of the newer single-chip cameras (Figure 4.1) at a lower cost and usually with higher reliability than three-chip systems.

Picture quality also depends on more subjective aspects than resolution, such as colour balance and warmth. These are determined by the image processing involved and to some extent the light source.

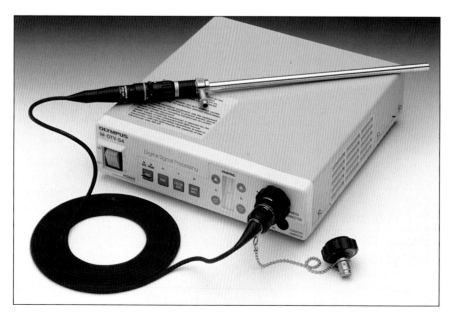

Figure 4.1 *Olympus OTV-S4 camera system (courtesy of KeyMed (Medical & Industrial Equipment) Ltd, Southend-on-Sea, UK).*

Light source

A high-power light source is essential. Although a satisfactory view may be obtained most of the time with inferior quality equipment, blood absorbs the light in a very dramatic fashion so that as soon as any bleeding occurs the image may become unusable at the very time when it is most important to be able to see clearly.

It is preferable that the camera and light source are from the same manufacturer so that they can communicate to adjust brightness to avoid flare and white-out. A range of different light sources is available; the xenon sources generally have brighter illumination than the halogen ones (Figure 4.2). Others are likely to be developed in due course.

In general terms, the more one pays the more powerful the light source is likely to be. However, a further variable which needs to be considered is the life expectancy of the bulb and whether it can be replaced by the user or must be returned to the manufacturer for replacement: some cheaper units have greater running costs. Ideally, a cold light source or one with an infrared filter should be chosen to avoid the risk of burning the patient or damaging the endoscope. With these facts in mind, and within the limits of hospital budget policy on capital equipment purchase and maintenance or revenue costs, you should carefully review the equipment available within your price range, clarifying with the manufacturers their policy about replacement instruments and maintenance contracts.

Endoscopes

Endoscopes (Figure 4.3) have a finite life in a busy operating theatre. With repeated soaking or autoclaving they deteriorate, with the result that the image is degraded. Ideally, endoscopes should be replaced

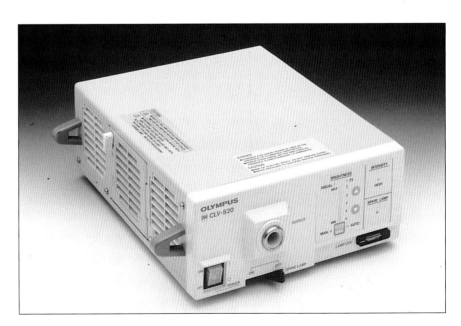

Figure 4.2 *Olympus CLV-S20 light source. This light source has a 300 W xenon light bulb (courtesy of KeyMed (Medical & Industrial Equipment) Ltd, Southend-on-Sea, UK).*

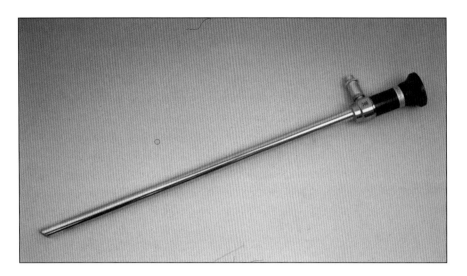

Figure 4.3 *Olympus OES autoclavable laparoscope (courtesy of KeyMed (Medical & Industrial Equipment) Ltd, Southend-on-Sea, UK).*

every year because the loss of image quality is insidious and often not noticed by day-to-day users. A good camera system is unable to make up for old endoscopes.

The most commonly used laparoscope for gynaecological endoscopy is the 10 mm 0° scope. These instruments use the Hopkins rod lens systems. Smaller endoscopes give a reduced field of view and substantially reduced passage of light, and are not generally suitable for operative laparoscopy.

The most commonly used hysteroscopes are between 3 and 4 mm in diameter and have a 30° objective lens which enables inspection of the uterine cornua. Even smaller scopes are in use for outpatient hysteroscopy (Figure 4.4) The decreased illumination is not such a problem in the uterus because the cavity is smaller and there is less dissipation of light than at laparoscopy.

An operative laparoscope with an offset viewing channel and concentric 5 mm instrument channel (Figure 4.5) is used with the carbon dioxide laser and has the advantage of being able to accept a

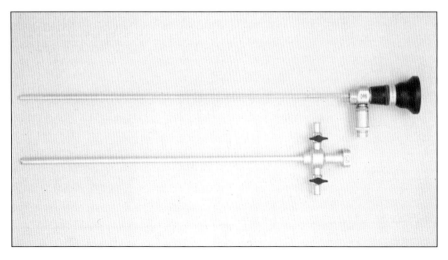

Figure 4.4 *Olympus OES autoclavable 3 mm hysteroscope (courtesy of KeyMed (Medical & Industrial Equipment) Ltd, Southend-on-Sea, UK).*

Figure 4.5 *Olympus CO_2 Lasercoupler system (courtesy of KeyMed (Medical & Industrial Equipment) Ltd, Southend-on-Sea, UK).*

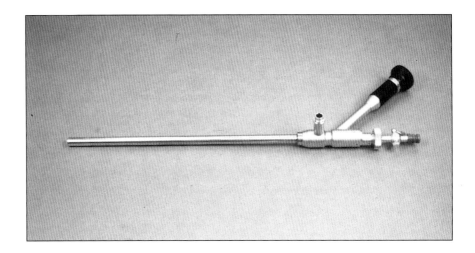

5 mm instrument when not connected to the laser. However, there is a substantial loss of image quality and illumination.

Recently, a lot of attention has been focused on small-diameter laparoscopy using scopes of around 2 mm in diameter. These have the advantage of being able to pass through a Veress needle, and can be used in alternative insufflation sites to ensure that the primary trocar insertion site is free from adhesions. Their place in operative laparoscopy is otherwise very limited.

Other new developments include the mounting of the video chip on the end of a 10 mm diameter probe, thus eliminating the need for the rod lens system and powerful light sources. These instruments are not widely available at present but may have a large impact on future instrument design.

Most laparoscopes are reusable, although a single-use model is available (Auto Suture, Ascot, UK). The usual standards for cleaning and sterilization apply. Most manufacturers have models that can be autoclaved, although previously glutaraldehyde-based cleansing solutions were the most commonly used means of sterilizing instruments between cases. The risks associated with glutaraldehyde and its potential toxicity are well known, and most hospitals are trying to cut down on its use. With long-term use, glutaraldehyde is also damaging to instruments. It is particularly important to make a decision about the method of sterilization at the time of purchase and not to change the selected method, because autoclaving instruments that have previously been soaked in glutaraldehyde, or vice versa, is particularly damaging.

The camera should never be soaked in glutaraldehyde solutions. It is the author's practice to use a sterile polyethylene sheath for the camera, and to autoclave the laparoscopes and light connection cable. Others prefer to wipe the camera and light cable with an alcohol-soaked swab.

Carbon dioxide insufflator

A number of excellent insufflators (Figure 4.6) are available from all the major instrument manufacturers. It is essential to have an insufflator capable of providing a flow rate of at least 9 l/min. Flows of this rate are required to replace gas lost at instrument removal or specimen retrieval. It is important that the insufflator can be pressure regulated separately from the rate of flow. Most now have digital light-emitting diode (LED) indicators showing the pressure setting and flow rate. Some instruments also have gas heaters and humidifiers built into the instrument.

Carbon dioxide is the most commonly used distension medium for laparoscopy. Helium and nitrous oxide (N_2O) have also been used successfully. Nitric oxide (NO) should not be used for operative laparoscopy because it forms a potentially explosive mixture with oxygen.

Gasless laparoscopy

The use of pneumatic and simple mechanical lifting bars introduced through incisions in the anterior abdominal wall to provide exposure without the creation of a pneumoperitoneum has been described. The stated advantages are that exposure can be achieved without splinting the diaphragm, and there is no tamponade of small vessels causing unrecognized haemorrhage after surgery, or loss of exposure when the vagina is opened during laparoscopically assisted vaginal hysterectomy or posterior colpotomy. However, they do cause considerable trauma to the peritoneum of the anterior abdominal wall.

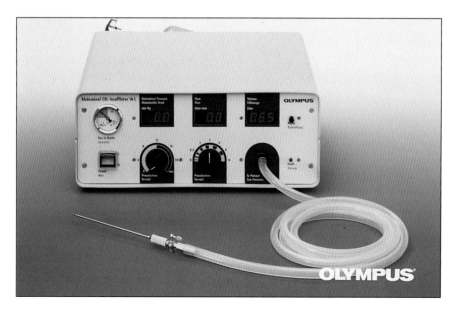

Figure 4.6 *Olympus CO_2 insufflator, producing a flow rate of 0.5–16 l/min (courtesy of KeyMed (Medical & Industrial Equipment) Ltd, Southend-on-Sea, UK).*

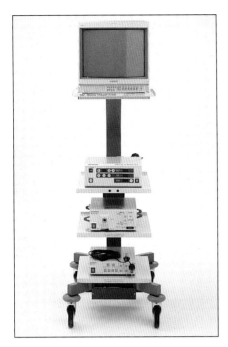

Figure 4.7 *KeyMed laparoscopic surgery instrument trolley (courtesy of KeyMed (Medical & Industrial Equipment) Ltd, Southend-on-Sea, UK).*

Theatre layout

It is most convenient for all the imaging equipment and the insufflator to be placed on a purpose-built trolley with the monitor (Figure 4.7). All the instruments are then readily visible to the lead surgeon.

The operating theatre layouts preferred by the author for most gynaecological procedures are shown in Figures 4.8 and 4.9. The first assistant acts as camera operator and uses the second monitor. A Mayo table over the patient's head can be useful, as can an instrument tray placed on the end of the table, between the patient's legs, for laparoscopically assisted vaginal hysterectomy.

Suction/irrigation equipment

This piece of equipment is among the most useful, ensuring adequate exposure in the presence of haemorrhage. The irrigation probe can be used to introduce a contact laser fibre, to aspirate smoke or fluid, or to irrigate with clear saline or the more physiological Hartmann's solution. The probe is also used for blunt dissection and aquadissection. A number of methods of pressurizing the irrigation fluid are available, including roller pumps, positive pressure pumps using air or carbon dioxide insufflated into rigid bottles containing irrigation fluid, and arterial pressure infusion pumps placed around standard Baxter infusion bags. In the author's experience the most

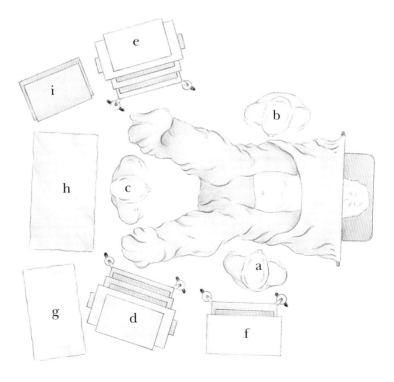

Figure 4.8 *Operating theatre layout with one assistant. (a) Lead surgeon, (b) assistant, (c) nurse, (d) video stack, (e) stack 1, (f) stack 2, (g) D & C trolley, (h) back table, (i) diathermy generator.*

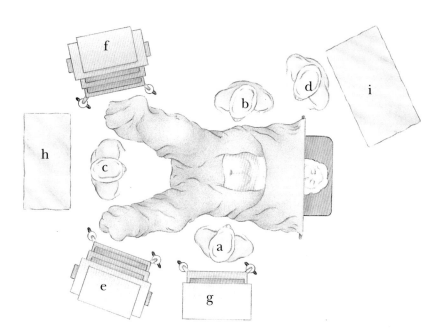

Figure 4.9 *Operating theatre layout with two assistants. (a) Lead surgeon, (b) first assistant, (c) second assistant, (d) nurse, (e) video stack, (f) stack 1, (g) stack 2, (h) D & C trolley, (i) back table.*

efficient is the Cabot Niagara pump (Corey Bros., London, UK; Figure 4.10). This consists of a rigid box with an inflatable balloon membrane on one side, which is connected to the anaesthetic gas supply. The pressure in the balloon is regulated but adjustable, and remains constant regardless of the volume of fluid in the bag. This irrigation system, combined with standard vacuum suction equipment, works most effectively. Cabot also manufacture a disposable tubing and valve set (Figure 4.11) to which can be attached a range of reusable probes of 5 and 10 mm diameter. The larger diameter probes can carry a 5 mm instrument; both sizes can accommodate a laser fibre.

Access

The range of trocars and cannulae available is vast. The commonly used sizes are 5, 10 and 12 mm in diameter. A variety of valve mechanisms is available, ranging from no valve at all to flap valves or trumpet valves. The flap valves are easier to use as they do not grasp the shaft of instruments; trumpet valves do, and this can prove most irritating as the trocars are often inadvertently pulled out when the instruments stick. More importantly, trumpet valves can strip the insulation off the shaft of electrosurgical instruments, leading to potentially dangerous leakage of electrical energy to the trocar. Trumpet valves were popular because they could easily be held open to allow gas and smoke to escape or tissue to be removed, but new designs have overcome this problem and most flap valves now also include a means of holding the valve open.

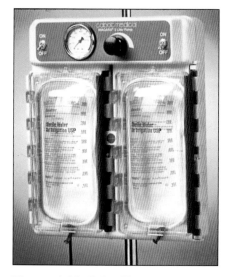

Figure 4.10 *Cabot Niagara 2L irrigation pump (courtesy of Cabot Medical, Langhorne, USA).*

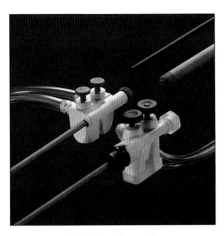

Figure 4.11 *Cabot Surgiflex suction/irrigation probe (courtesy of Cabot Medical, Langhorne, USA).*

Most single-use and some reusable trocars have guard mechanisms to protect the pelvic organs from the sharp trocar once the peritoneum has been breached. These are really relevant only for the first trocar insertion, as all others should be made under direct vision. Even for a first puncture their usefulness has not been conclusively demonstrated.

Port closure

Where cannulae larger than 10 mm in diameter are used, the sheath should be closed to prevent hernia formation. This can be particularly difficult in all but the slimmest of patients unless appropriate needles and instruments are used. Among the simplest and most effective is the Phipps J-shaped needle (Rocket, London, UK; Figure 4.12). This is inserted into the abdominal cavity under direct vision and used to close the peritoneum sheath and subcutaneous fatty tissue in a simple loop, thus eliminating the chance of hernia formation.

Endoscopic surgical instruments

A wide range of hand instruments is available, including atraumatic and traumatic grasping forceps, scissors, needle holders, clamps and diathermy probes, again in both reusable or single-use forms. Trainee surgeons will become familiar with the instruments used by their trainers. As their experience increases, they will develop preferences of their own. The important features to consider are ease of dismantling for cleaning, robust design and precision engineering. The length of the instrument should feel comfortable: the usual length is about 30 cm, which is about right when inserted through the cannula, although this does feel uncomfortable when not so supported. Longer instruments are available for use in the central channel of operating laparoscopes. These are less easy to use through secondary cannulae.

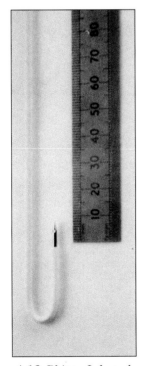

Figure 4.12 *Phipps J-shaped needle. (Reproduced from* Gynaecological Endoscopy *1994; 3: 190 with permission from Blackwell Science Ltd., Oxford, UK).*

Tissue extraction

Tissue can be removed through the anterior abdominal wall or through the posterior fornix, using either retrieval bags or tissue morcellators or a combination. The anterior abdominal wall is the site of choice for small specimens such as fallopian tube or biopsy specimens. However, the rectus sheath is relatively inelastic and tissue of greater than 10 mm in diameter will require an enlarged incision in the sheath; this can be tricky to close and has an associated risk of hernia formation. The posterior fornix is a useful site for tissue extraction. The problem of loss of pneumoperitoneum pressure can be overcome by using the CCL vaginal extraction kit (Storz, Tuttlingen, Germany) (Figure 4.13). This is essentially a flap valve trocar mechanism with an insulated ball at the distal end, which both distends the posterior fornix and forms a seal with the skin of the vagina. Diathermy or laser is used to cut down onto the ball, thus opening the elastic skin of the posterior fornix. Large specimens can be retrieved with ease by introducing a 10 mm grasping forceps through the cannula and removing the specimen either with or without a bag.

One of the simplest retrieval bags to use is the EndoCatch (Auto Suture, Ascot, UK) (Figure 4.14). This has a bag attached to a spring steel rim which automatically holds the bag open while the specimen is introduced.

Specimens that are too large to be retrieved in this fashion can be reduced in size using a tissue morcellator. A number of mechanisms exist for this, from simply cutting the specimen up with scissors or diathermy, through a range of instruments that effectively core out tissue. The most sophisticated of these is the Steiner morcellator (Storz; Figure 4.15), which is motor driven and can remove a 6 × 8 cm uterus or fibroid through a 12 mm cannula in about 5 min.

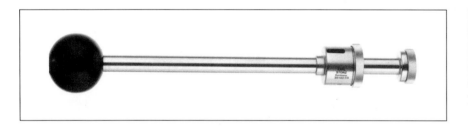

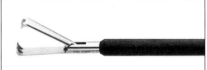

Figure 4.13 *CCL vaginal extraction kit (courtesy of Karl Storz GmbH & Co., Tuttlingen, Germany).*

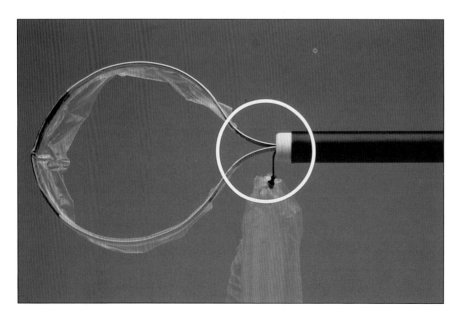

Figure 4.14 *Endocatch tissue retrieval bag (courtesy of Auto Suture Company, Ascot UK).*

Figure 4.15 *Steiner tissue morcellator. (courtesy of Karl Storz GmbH & Co., Tuttlingen, Germany).*

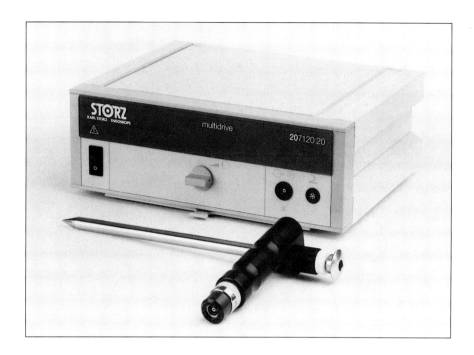

Electrosurgical generators

A modern electrosurgical generator is an important and highly versatile part of the endoscopic surgeon's equipment. It should have both bipolar and unipolar capabilities and display the power generated in watts. Some modern instruments detect the degree of desiccation achieved and automatically adjust the power settings to avoid charring and unnecessary heating of tissue. There is no doubt that in skilled hands the electrosurgical generator can be a most versatile and effective instrument. However, it should be remembered that inappropriate use of electrosurgery has been responsible for a number of disastrous accidents.

Bipolar coagulation

Bipolar coagulation provides a relatively safe and efficient means of arresting haemorrhage, and should be immediately available in all endoscopic surgical procedures. A range of jaw sizes and shapes is available. The simplest and most versatile is the 3 mm wide straight spring closing variety.

Safety point

Inappropriate use of electrosurgery can cause disastrous accidents.

Lasers

The use of lasers is described in Chapter 16.

Other instruments

There are a number of other instruments available which offer alternative means of achieving safe haemostasis, cutting or vaporization of tissue, including the harmonic scalpel, argon beam coagulator, and combined bipolar forceps and cutting instruments, as well as alternative forms of clips and staples. These will not be discussed further in this book. Once trainee surgeons have developed a high degree of skill with conventional laparoscopic instruments, they will be in a position to judge the usefulness or otherwise of alternative instruments.

Summary

The surgeon and his team must be familiar with their equipment and its vagaries. In the event of unexpected equipment failure replacement equipment should be in a state of readiness for immediate use and easily accessible. The layout of the equipment in particular the video monitors should be arranged in accordance with the lead surgeon's requirements. All members of the team, surgeons, nurses and technicians should be trained to be familiar with all the equipment as the success of the surgery is dependent on team-work. There is a greater requirement for circulating nurses and theatre technicians than in conventional surgery.

Chapter 5

Understanding Electrosurgery: Safety and Efficiency

J.H. Phipps

Introduction

This chapter explains basic radiofrequency (RF) physics in terms useful to the clinician. Understanding the behaviour of RF energy in biological tissues is of paramount importance, especially in endoscopic surgery, where it is essential to understand that the effects of applying such energy may not be limited to the surgical field; indeed, such application may exert effects that may seem incomprehensible without a good basic working knowledge.

Misconceptions

Mythology and misconceptions abound whenever diathermy is discussed. 'Never use monopolar diathermy in the abdomen'[1] is a widely stated dogma with little justification or basis in biophysical fact. 'Laser causes so much less scarring ...', again widely believed but not true[2,3]. Professor Soderstrom's 'a watt is a Watt is a Watt'[4] at the cellular level is apposite, but appreciated by few. It is my hope that the few words in this chapter will stay in the minds of endoscopic surgeons. Following the basic principles outlined here will, without doubt, reduce complications, including danger to the surgeon and, in certain situations, life itself.

Terminology

The term 'diathermy' was coined in the early part of the century for the application of RF energy to heat the deep tissues of the pelvis for the treatment of gonorrhoea (*Neisseria* species are very heat sensitive). For present purposes, however, 'diathermy' refers to the application of RF energy for surgical cutting and/or coagulation of tissues.

'Fulguration' is the application of high voltage (that is, 'coagulation current') to an area of bleeding using a no-touch technique. This allows sparking (arcing) to occur between the electrode and the target tissue (of which more later), for the purpose of securing haemostasis. A good example of this is the use of ball diathermy after large diathermy loop excision of the cervical transformation zone. Fulguration is merely one physical method of applying coagulation, and will not be discussed further because the principles underlying its use are the same as for coagulation phenomena in general.

Diathermy has been used for over 50 years, and relies on the properties of the passage of RF current at (typically) a frequency of around 500 kHz through biological tissues. The result of current flow through tissues is heating, and the exact method used to induce this heating determines the surgical effect obtained (i.e. warming, coagulation or cutting of tissue). The rationale for using this frequency is that current flowing through tissues at much under 100 kHz causes contraction of muscle and cellular depolarization, which produces the phenomenon known as electrocution. At 500 kHz (a commonly used frequency) and above, however, the voltage across the individual cell changes its polarity so quickly that the ionic shifts across the cell membrane which facilitate muscle contraction do not have time to occur. Electrocution does not, therefore, occur when current frequency is very high (as in modern diathermy). Direct application of diathermy to muscle, however, does cause contraction, as any surgeon is aware. This is caused by both 'impurities' in the signal from the diathermy generator and alterations in the signal ('demodulation') such that lower-frequency harmonics of the signal are produced (i.e. some of the current flowing is below 100 kHz).

Diathermy generators produce essentially three basic modes of output: monopolar cutting current, monopolar coagulation current, and so-called 'bipolar' current. The differences between, and the advantages and disadvantages of, bipolar diathermy are discussed below. The general principles and mode of action of diathermy are best illustrated by a consideration of the monopolar mode first.

Monopolar diathermy

The difference between cutting and coagulation output is one of waveform. Diagrammatically represented, cutting current is a relatively low-amplitude continuous sine wave, where the x-axis represents voltage and the y-axis time (Figure 5.1).

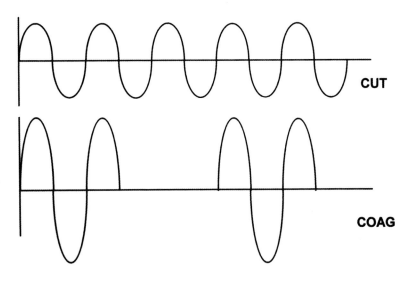

Figure 5.1 *Cutting and coagulation waveforms.*

The biological effect of this type of signal in sufficiently high volume and current density at the point of contact with tissue (of which more later) is a very rapid increase in temperature to the extent that the target tissue vaporizes, and the surgeon sees a cutting effect. Coagulation waveforms are more complex and vary from machine to machine, but all have in common an on–off–on waveform, where the signal is chopped such that, in cumulative terms, the current is more off than on (Figure 5.1). The amplitude (voltage) of the coagulation signal (when in 'on' mode) is higher than that for cutting. The biological effect of this type of waveform, when applied in exactly the same way as the cutting current, i.e. with an identical surface area of contact with tissue, is to rapidly heat the tissue momentarily during the 'on' phase but allow sufficient time to cool during the 'off' phase, so that tissue does not vaporize, and thermal 'spread' is allowed to occur. The surgeon sees 'coagulation'. The two signals may be mixed to provide an effect that combines coagulation and cutting (blended current).

The signal strength and waveform are not the only factors that determine the final biological effect. Another, usually more important, factor – that of surface area of contact of the applicator (usually a surgical instrument) with the tissue – also plays a major part.

Tissue effects of radiofrequency energy

The voltage applied to tissue in electrosurgery is alternating, therefore the current that flows as a result of the voltage being applied is also alternating, at about 500 kHz. To the electrical engineer, the patient may be represented by a resistor and a capacitor, wired together in parallel, which may be referred to as the electrical load (Figure 5.2). Because the body acts as both a resistor and a capacitor, current flowing at diathermy-type frequency (i.e. about 500 kHz) is able to do so both through the resistive electrical component of the body and through the capacitative component. Although non-alternating electrical current (direct current, or DC) is unable to pass through a capacitor, alternating current (AC) is able to pass by rapidly changing the polarity of the charge on either side of the capacitor, which leads to a flow of electrons across the capacitor, and therefore current flow. This concept is important, as we shall see.

The overall ability of the body or tissues to resist or 'impede' the passage of diathermy current is called impedance. A high tissue impedance means that relatively little current is able to flow through a given structure or volume of tissue (for example, a heat-desiccated pedicle), and a low impedance implies the reverse.

It is an intrinsic property of RF energy at diathermy frequencies that the majority of current passes resistively, i.e. only a small proportion of the total current flow passes as a result of the capacitance of the tissue. This is of great importance to the surgeon. The concept of current flow (and therefore heating) through tissues

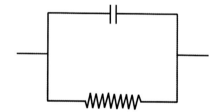

Figure 5.2 *Diagrammatic representation of a patient in electrical engineering terms.*

without apparent direct electrical contact is one that many find difficult, but it may cause considerable problems (see below).

The surgeon is interested not in current flow but in what happens at the end of the surgical instrument. The answer is, of course, heating. Although I have tried hard to refrain from putting equations in this chapter for fear of provoking dismissal from readers, I plead necessity for those of Ohm (whose application here, for the serious scientist, is limited because they take no account of capacitative phenomena, but for present purposes serve well):

$$V = IR$$

$$P = IV$$

where V is the voltage in volts, I the current in amperes, R the resistance in ohms, and P the power in watts. It requires only elementary algebra to manipulate these two simple equations to explain a great deal about the way diathermy heats tissue. For simplicity's sake, let us assume that P is proportional to the degree of heating of the target tissues (although in reality the relationship is not so exact or simple). The amount of heating, then, is a product of the voltage applied (V) and the current flowing (I). Let us further assume that the voltage is relatively fixed (that is, set by the output of the diathermy machine). The amount of heating is therefore directly proportional to the amount of current flowing. Going back to the first equation, $V = IR$, it is easy to see that $I = V/R$. If V is fixed, I is inversely proportional to R. In other words, the higher the tissue resistance (remember, we are for the present ignoring the capacitative qualities of tissue), the lower the current flowing, and the lower the degree of heating.

So current flow in tissues causes heating. The biological effects of this are irreversible destruction of cells by denaturation of vital proteins and desiccation. This may be to an extreme and rapid degree, where tissue heating is such that the surgeon sees electrosurgical cutting (i.e. cellular vaporization), or to a slower more diffuse pattern, producing electrosurgical coagulation. This sounds obvious, but the story does not end there. There is a third type of biologically relevant heating, whose effects are not apparent at the time of surgery, but manifest some 48–72 h later: those of hyperthermia. Mammalian cells are capable of surviving heating to approximately 42°C but, at higher temperatures, irreversible damage occurs which is dependent on both time of exposure and temperature. Irreversible denaturation of cytoskeletal proteins is the first morbid event to occur, and begins after about 60 min at 42°C. Such thermotolerance time is approximately halved for every degree rise in temperature[5] (Figure 5.3).

Immediate effects of such heating are subtle, and cannot be detected by histological examination or enzyme degradation studies if

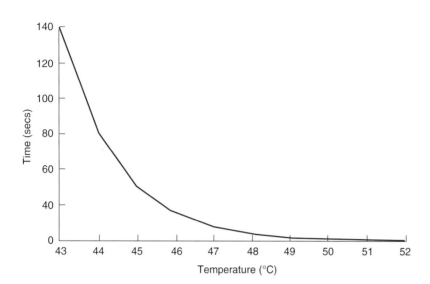

Figure 5.3 *Thermotolerance time for mammalian cells* in vitro.

looked for immediately after exposure[6]. Hyperthermic tissue damage is often not taken into account when mapping thermal destruction after tissue exposure to diathermy heating[7], leading to potential overestimation of safety. For example, cases of bowel injury after intrauterine electrosurgery have been reported on a number of occasions[8], although no overt penetration of the myometrium occurred. Such cases are almost certainly due to hyperthermic tissue damage rather than straightforward burns. Thermal spread beyond the range immediately apparent at the time of surgery must always be borne in mind.

Area of surface contact, field effect and current density

One of the most important concepts to grasp about diathermy is that, despite the previous handling of current flow and heating along simple Ohm's law principles, we are not dealing with simple resistive current flow when it comes to considering how diathermy behaves clinically. It is at this point that we must draw the line to 'hard' physics and accept that a number of statements about RF energy are true, without exploring the physical and mathematical corroborations that exist.

RF displays properties of field effect, typical of electromagnetic phenomena. In practical terms, flow of RF energy does not simply obey Ohm's law, but rather behaves as a field of energy whose flow pattern is determined to a large extent by the nature of the conductor–conductor interface (for present purposes, usually an interface between the diathermy-armed surgical instrument and the target tissue). 'RF loves edges and corners' is an old saying of radio transmitter engineers, and for the surgeon to understand this statement is of paramount importance. The surgeon who comes to appreciate this will be more able to use diathermy safely and efficiently. Explanation requires several examples.

The interface between the diathermy applicator and the tissues becomes heated, but the interface between the patient and the return electrode plate does not, because of the different surface areas of contact. The area of contact at the return electrode plate is many thousand times greater than that of the instrument–tissue area of contact, and the current density between the two is correspondingly high. The same current clearly has to flow between the diathermy instrument and the point of tissue contact as between the return plate and the patient's leg (Figure 5.4), but the surface area across which that current has to flow is much smaller at the point of tissue contact. The concept of current density is very important to the surgeon. Anyone who uses diathermy in open surgery will have noticed that the smaller the area of contact of the diathermy forceps with the tissue, the faster and more extreme the heating effect. If diathermy forceps are held in contact with tissue in such a way that the whole of the exposed tip of the forceps is in contact, it becomes very difficult to heat and cauterize the tissue at all. This is a function of current density.

For the endoscopic surgeon, this phenomenon may be used to good effect when cutting and dissecting tissues using laparoscopic instruments. Many instruments afford the surgeon the ability to create a relatively large surface area of contact with tissue when held in one particular position, such that current density is relatively low when the instrument is activated, but the area of contact is smaller when applied in another position with a correspondingly higher current density. In the former position, the instrument effectively coagulates tissue, but in

Figure 5.4 *Current flow in monopolar diathermy. The area of surface contact is large between the return electrode and the patient, hence the current density and therefore the heating are very low. The reverse is true for the interface between the active instrument tip and the target tissue.* $I_1 = I_2$; *heating is inversely proportional to area of surface contact.*

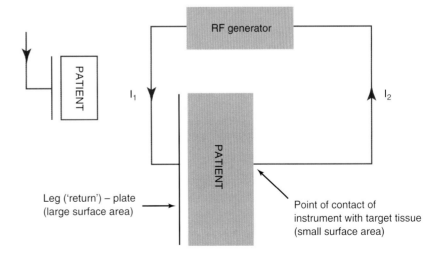

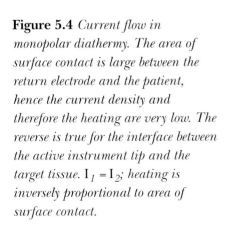

$I_1 = I_2$ – heating is inversely proportional to area of surface contact

the position of small area of surface contact the instrument becomes an effective cutting tool. The most obvious example of such an instrument is the flat diathermy hook, but scissors (which may be used to cut or, with the blades closed, as a flat cauterizing surface) are another example. This works to the advantage of the surgeon who is aware of the current density phenomenon. On the other hand, the surgeon who repeatedly attempts to stem bleeding from a leaking vessel using the tip of an instrument rather than its flat wide surface, will be rewarded with increasing haemorrhage as the high current density of the diathermy application leads to more and more tissue vaporization (a common mistake).

Appreciation of current density phenomena is even more important when one considers 'stray' diathermy. The potential for high current density on any RF-charged surface will be marked wherever there is an edge or a corner on that charged surface. I am not suggesting that this experiment should be tried, but if the surgeon touches an RF-live surface, such as the exposed output pin of the diathermy generator (at low output) in a bold manner, so that the whole of the surface of the fingers is in contact with the pin, the experimenter will feel very little or nothing. On the other hand, gingerly touching the pin with the very tip of a finger will cause current to begin to flow via a very small surface area, and shock will result.

Finally, in practical terms, the surgeon should bear in mind that a far more significant factor in determining whether a particular diathermy application cuts or coagulates is area of surface contact, not whether a cutting or a coagulating waveform is applied.

Bipolar diathermy

This type of diathermy has become very popular in recent years, and is said to be much safer than monopolar by many surgical authorities, with some justification, although there are qualifications that must be borne in mind.

The essential difference between the two modes is that in bipolar diathermy both arms of the circuit are delivered to the surgical instrument (usually grasping forceps) and no return electrode plate needs to be attached to the patient (Figure 5.5). The great advantage of this is that current flow is largely limited exclusively to the surgical field, because the two jaws of the bipolar instrument are live only with respect to one another. However, under certain circumstances, each jaw of the forceps (especially when activated with no tissue interposed between them) may be live with respect to surrounding tissues[9]. It is therefore a point of safety that, in common with all applications of diathermy, the instrument must *never* be activated inside the abdomen without good contact with target tissue. This is especially important with monopolar diathermy (see below). The reason for this is that,

Figure 5.5 *(a) Bipolar and (b) monopolar current flow.*

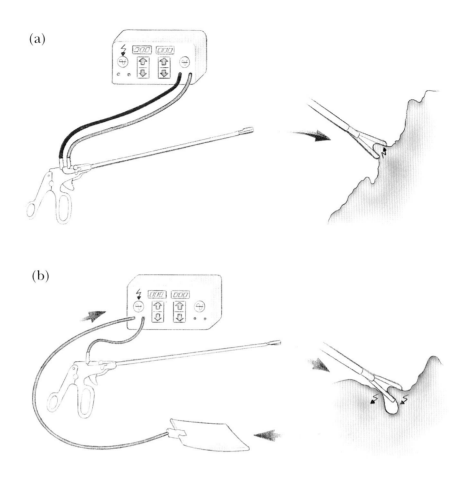

unless the activated diathermy-armed tip of the instrument is in good contact with target tissue, a high voltage exists between the instrument and the surrounding non-target tissue (notably bowel), with consequent risk of stray current flow and burns.

The effect of passing current across tissues in such a way is, again, heating. Bipolar diathermy is therefore confined largely to coagulation. (Although there are instruments which purport to cut using bipolar diathermy, these tend to be of limited efficiency at present). Although it lacks the flexibility of monopolar diathermy, the bipolar mode is unquestionably safer in certain respects.

It should be borne in mind, however, that tissue heated with bipolar diathermy becomes very hot indeed (around 340°C at the

Safety point

A diathermy instrument must **never** be activated without good contact with the target tissue.

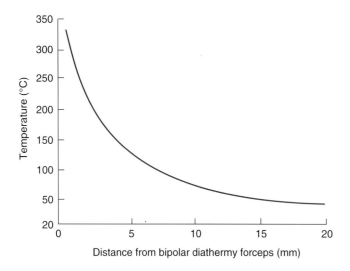

Figure 5.6 *Temperature* versus *distance from epicentre of bipolar diathermy application.*

point of maximal current flow), such that a significant thermal gradient is driven by such heating (Figure 5.6). After 8 s of bipolar diathermy application, tissue as distant as 15 mm may be heated to levels[10] sufficient to cause tissue damage, simply by thermal spread.

Hazards of electrosurgery

The dangers of using RF electrical energy in surgery are the subject of increasing interest, and are now commonly cited in medicolegal cases. It is therefore of paramount importance that anyone using RF electrosurgery (not only surgeons) is knowledgeable about relevant theory and practicalities.

There are a number of ways to categorize hazards associated with diathermy use, but the following seems logical.

Conductive thermal gradients
Diathermy application leads to heating of a sometimes unsuspected degree and extent. It should be borne in mind that histotoxic spread of heat will always be considerably beyond the tissue boundaries demarked by simple observation of whitening of tissue.

Most hazards associated with diathermy are, however, electrical (Figure 5.7).

Direct coupling
The most obvious and common surgical error committed with diathermy is the accidental heating of tissue that is not the intended target (non-target tissue). Accidental heating of non-target tissue may occur as a result of two major variable factors.

The first is the proximity of non-target tissue to the operative site. Clearly, if diathermy is applied to a target structure that lies

Figure 5.7 *Potential causes of unwanted heating and burns, beyond the field of vision of the surgeon, due to stray current flow.*

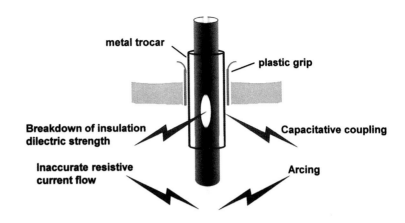

anatomically very close to a non-target structure (e.g. a bleeding pedicle lying adjacent to bowel), there is a risk that the non-target structure will be accidentally contacted by the diathermy-armed instrument, resulting in current flow, heating and non-target tissue necrosis[11].

The second issue is that of tissue impedance. The example of a bleeding pedicle adjacent to bowel serves well to illustrate this effect. When the diathermy instrument is applied to the bleeding pedicle and activated, the tissue impedance of the pedicle and the bowel to which it lies in close proximity are roughly equivalent. Current therefore flows exclusively through target tissue, and at this stage no problem arises. However, as heating of the pedicle proceeds, it becomes desiccated, its water content falls, and its impedance therefore rises. If diathermy is continued, current flow may occur through the adjacent non-target tissue because the impedance of the non-target tissue, which has not been desiccated, is much lower (Figure 5.8). This is the classic situation where arcing of diathermy current occurs to bowel when pelvic structures such as fallopian tubes are cauterized with monopolar diathermy.

Whenever monopolar diathermy is activated without a desirable earth pathway (i.e. through target tissue), especially with the high voltages used with coagulation mode, there is always a risk of unwanted current flow and arcing to non-target tissues. Devices now reaching the market may help to reduce such risks under certain circumstances, but we shall consider these in more detail under the heading of capacitative coupling.

Insulation failure

This is now rare as the quality of insulation used for instrument manufacture has improved; it almost never occurs if disposable instruments are used. Clearly, if insulation is damaged or inadequate

(a)

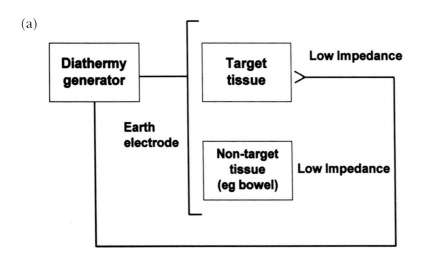

(b)

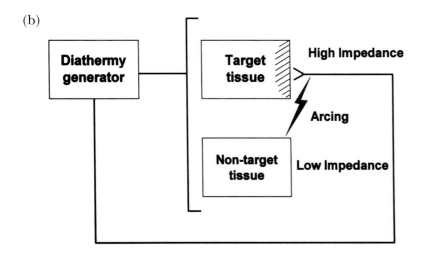

Figure 5.8 *(a) Flow of current from the active instrument tip into target tissue at the beginning of current flow, when the target tissue is still fully hydrated and therefore of low impedance. Current flows into the target tissue rather than into the immediately adjacent non-target tissue (e.g. a piece of bowel) because the impedances of the two at this stage are identical and the instrument tip is closer to the target tissue than to the non-target tissue. (b) Current flow after target tissue heating and desiccation. The impedance of the non-target tissue is now much lower compared with the desiccated target tissue. If the non-target tissue is very close to the instrument tip, current may preferentially flow to non-target tissue and cause burns.*

around the diathermy charged core of an instrument, there is a risk of current leakage from the instrument either to other instruments (such as cannulae) or, worse, to non-target tissues. Insulation failure most commonly occurs when the insulation at the terminal end of a laparoscopic instrument is cracked and peels away from the conductive core such that arcing to non-target tissue close to the operative site occurs. It is worth noting that faulty insulation may not be visible. It must be borne in mind that diathermy uses relatively high voltages,

Safety point

It is vitally important that monopolar diathermy never be activated without good contact of the instrument tip with target tissue.

particularly in coagulation mode. The ability of any insulating material to resist current leakage is termed its dielectric strength. When insulating material is repeatedly heated and cooled during sterilization its dielectric strength is invariably degraded to some extent, with consequent risk of unwanted leakage and arcing even if the insulation is macroscopically intact.

Capacitative coupling

This phenomenon has received a great deal of attention recently, but the risks of patient injury related to the effect have probably been exaggerated provided the surgeon is aware that capacitative coupling exists and follows the elementary steps required to prevent any such problems.

Capacitative coupling occurs as the result of RF current flowing through one conductor (the conductive core of the diathermy instrument) which is separated from another conductor (the metal sheath of the cannula) by an insulating material (the coating of the diathermy instrument). The system acts as a capacitor, with the insulating coat around the core of the diathermy instrument acting as the dielectric. Charge is therefore induced in the metal cannula body without direct contact with any conductive charged surface. Provided that the metal cannula is in good electrical contact with the abdominal wall such charge is harmlessly dispersed into the abdominal wall. Because of the large area of contact of the metal cannula with the abdominal wall tissues, current density is very low and heating is negligible. However, if the metal cannula first passes through a plastic collar in the abdominal wall, such that it is insulated from the abdominal wall, any induced charge in the metal cannula body will not be dispersed because the cannula is electrically isolated. It is therefore possible that the metal cannula effectively becomes live every time the diathermy instrument passing through it is activated. The worst possible scenario is that during this episode a small area of bowel will be touching the metal cannula and, obviously, outside the field of laparoscopic vision. If the area of contact of bowel with cannula is sufficiently small, the charged cannula will earth itself through the bowel with correspondingly high current density, and a burn will result[12,13] (Figure 5.9). The phenomenon may be responsible for visceral injuries apparently remote from the operative site.

Two simple measures (summarized below) will reduce the risks associated with capacitative coupling virtually to zero. First, metal cannulae must never be used with plastic collars (gripping devices). If metal cannulae are employed, conductive metal collars must be used. These allow any charge induced in the metal cannula to be harmlessly dispersed through the abdominal wall. Alternatively, all-plastic cannulae may be employed, which removes the risk altogether. The second precaution has already been forcefully stated: never activate the

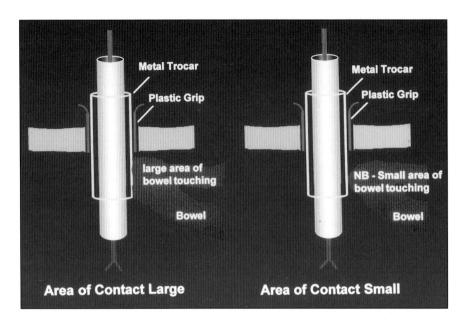

Figure 5.9 *Capacitative coupling. The metal cannula may become live every time the instrument passing down its centre is activated, because it is sited through the abdominal wall via a plastic (insulating) skin grip. If the area of contact of bowel with the cannula is small, the current density as the energy flows to earth will be high and a bowel burn will result. This problem can be completely eliminated by using only plastic grips with plastic cannulae and only metal grips with metal cannulae. Plastic cannulae without special earthing strips must never be used with uninsulated instruments inside the abdomen such as washer–sucker devices and laparoscopes.*

diathermy under 'open circuit' conditions. Activation of the monopolar diathermy without adequate desirable earthing (i.e. through target tissue) leads to very high voltages between the conductive core of the diathermy instrument and the rest of the patient and also the cannula body. Such high voltages drive a larger capacitative current flow; the charge built up in the metal cannula may be substantial and the risks of capacitative coupling resulting in burns are higher.

Precautions to reduce the risks of capacitative coupling

- Never use metal cannulae with plastic collars
- Never activate the diathermy under 'open circuit' conditions

---

There is now a device on the market (Electroshield, Boulder, Colorado, USA) that forms an isolated conductive sheath around diathermy-armed instruments and detects any insulation failure, whether it be direct resistive current leakage (faulty insulation) or capacitative coupling. The shield is connected to a detection apparatus, which is linked to the diathermy generator to sense any current leakage and cut off the diathermy current. The major limitation with such a device is that discrimination between normal functioning and current leakage may be difficult.

When coagulation current is applied in relatively large volumes, the electroshield device may identify the consequent (normal) capacitative current flow from the instrument as a fault and shut the diathermy generator down. This can be very inconvenient for the surgeon, especially when faced with significant bleeding that requires immediate control. The second problem with such a device is that current leakage is detected only over that portion of the diathermy instrument covered by the detector shield. For example, current leakage from the distal end of the instrument will not be detected. Provided that metal cannulae are never used with plastic collars, problems arising as a result of capacitative coupling do not occur. Faulty insulation is rarely a problem provided good quality and/or disposable instruments are used. The most likely point on the instrument at which the mis-application of energy may cause problems is therefore at the distal end, and the most likely cause is failure of the surgeon to adequately discriminate and separate target from non-target tissue; this, of course, is not covered by the sensor shielding device. Future development of this technology, with the sensor shield integral with the instrument such that the entire length of the instrument is covered, may however make for safer operating.

Finally, if activation of the diathermy-armed instrument does not produce the expected effect inside the abdomen within a few seconds, the generator power must *never* be increased straight away. It is essential that all connections are double checked before concluding that diathermy power is inadequate. It is sobering to realise that the most common causes of failure of diathermy are power connection to the wrong instrument (such that the viscera are exposed to diathermy power without visual monitoring) and failure to connect the diathermy instrument at all. The latter may result in horrific injury to the patient; there has been at least one case of corneal burn caused by the exposed pin at the end of the diathermy cable lying on the patient's face while the surgeon stood on the pedal wondering why the diathermy was not cutting inside the abdomen.

Earth (return) electrodes

Most modern diathermy machines use earth electrodes which are virtually foolproof in that a contact-sensor mechanism is built in so that the machine becomes non-functional in the event of poor patient contact. Prior to the introduction of this type of alarm system, it was possible for poor patient contact to reduce the area of contact with the return electrode and therefore cause burns to the patient's leg because

---

Safety point

If activation of the diathermy-armed instrument does not produce the expected effect inside the abdomen within a few seconds, the generator power must **never** be increased immediately.

---

of correspondingly high current density. It is obviously good practice to always use a new electrode pad, and place it on clean, dry, 'minimally hairy' skin.

Personnel and equipment safety

It is essential that both surgeon and paramedical theatre staff have a working knowledge of diathermy. It is beyond the scope of this chapter to describe in any detail safety protocols and theatre practice, but a sound working understanding of the physical principles governing the behaviour of electrosurgery equipment should underpin both of these. It is important that surgeons bear in mind that, ultimately, they are as responsible for the correct functioning of equipment when applied to the patient as the equipment manufacturer. All electrosurgical equipment has to conform to the rigorous standards laid out in the British Standard pertaining to electrical surgical equipment (BS 5724), but faults do occur. Clever design ensures that most faults 'fail safe', however, so that machine output is switched off if a problem does arise, although (as we have seen) this is by no means invariably the case. It is the responsibility of the surgeon, where this is reasonably possible, to make certain that the equipment is functioning correctly. For example, it would not be a reasonable defence for a surgeon to claim that the instrument manufacturers or the theatre staff were solely responsible for a bowel burn that resulted from damaged instrument insulation. It therefore behoves surgeons to make certain that they understand (to a reasonable and practicable degree) not only the theory behind the diathermy instruments but also the practical consequences of that theory.

Hazards to theatre staff (including the surgeon) are minimal under normal circumstances, but one or two points should be emphasized. The first is that the diathermy switch (pedal or handswitch) should *never* be activated until the theatre staff have finished connecting the machine properly. Surgical impatience has resulted in more than one operator's fingers receiving burns. RF burns are exceedingly painful and heal badly because of the penetrating nature of the injury.

A second common practice that should be abandoned is the casual use of metal (non-insulated) instruments to conduct diathermy to the surgical site. Typically, dissecting forceps are used for this to control small skin 'bleeders'. The bleeding tissue is picked up with the

Safety point

The surgeon is ultimately responsible for the correct functioning of electrosurgical equipment.

forceps, and the diathermy instrument is then activated in contact with the dissecting forceps. This should *never* be done. Most of the time, because the dissecting forceps are in good electrical contact with the patient, a good earth pathway is provided through target tissue. If, however, the surgeon slips and the diathermy (usually high-voltage coagulation current) is applied without good tissue contact, the voltage may find an earth pathway through the surgeon's fingers. If the insulation provided by the surgeon's glove breaks down, as it often does[14], a burn to the surgeon results.

Summary

Monopolar diathermy is the most flexible and powerful tool in the arsenal of the laparoscopic surgeon, and is cheap and widely available. The shift towards bipolar applications on the grounds that they are electrically safer is unfortunate. Bipolar diathermy by its very nature can never offer the same range of superb cutting and infinite variety of coagulative penetration that monopolar can. If monopolar diathermy is treated with understanding and respect, it is as safe, and probably safer, much more flexible, cheaper and more available than either bipolar systems or lasers. There is *nothing* that may be achieved with a laser in gynaecological surgery that cannot be performed with monopolar diathermy. It is simply a question of understanding the principle of varying the area of surface contact and therefore cutting density and which type of diathermy signal to apply. Even layer-by-layer stripping of the peritoneum over the ureter (often demonstrated as a task only achievable with laser) can easily be done with an ultrafine needle point with a low-voltage cutting waveform, with no difficulty at all. Electrosurgery has been with us for many years and, despite the intrusion of lasers, is again our mainstay when it comes to dealing with tissue division and haemostasis, and that is the way it is likely to stay.

References

1. Semm K (1983) Physical and biological considerations militating against the use of endoscopically applied high frequency current in the abdomen. *Endoscopy* **15**: 282–8.
2. Bordelon BM, Hobday KA, Hunter JG (1993) Laser *vs* electrosurgery in laparoscopic cholecystectomy: a prospective randomized trial. *Arch Surg* **128**: 233–6.
3. Palmer SE, McGill LD (1992) Thermal injury by *in vitro* incision of equine skin with electrosurgery, radiosurgery and a carbon dioxide laser. *Vet Surg* **21**: 348–50.

4. Soderstrom RM (1992) Electricity inside the uterus. *Clin Obstet Gynecol* **35**: 262–9.
5. Hahn GM (1982) *Hyperthermia and Cancer.* Springer-Verlag, New York, pp. 12–40.
6. Phipps JH (1992) Radiofrequency induced thermal endometrial ablation. MD thesis, University of Leicester.
7. Duffy S, Reid PC, Sharp F (1992) *In vivo* studies of uterine electrosurgery. *Br J Obstet Gynaecol* **99**: 579–82.
8. Sullivan B, Kenney P, Seibel M (1992) Hysteroscopic resection of fibroid with thermal injury to sigmoid colon. *Obstet Gynecol* **80**: 546–7.
9. Gilbert TB, Shaffer M, Matthews M (1991) Electrical shock by dislodged spark gap in bipolar electrosurgical device. *Anesth Analg* **73**: 355–7.
10. Phipps JH (1994) Thermometry studies with bipolar diathermy during hysterectomy. *Gynaecol Endosc* **3**: 5–7.
11. Ata AH, Bellemore TJ, Meisel JA, Arambulo SM (1993) Distal thermal injury from monopolar electrosurgery. *Surg Laparosc Endosc* **3**: 323–7.
12. Tucker RD, Voyles CR, Silvis SE (1992) Capacitive coupled stray currents during laparoscopic and endoscopic electrosurgical procedures. *Biomedical Instruments and Technology* **26**: 303–11.
13. Voyles CR, Tucker RD (1992) Education and engineering solutions for potential problems with laparoscopic monopolar electrosurgery. *Am J Surg* **146**: 57–62.
14. Tucker RD, Ferguson S (1991) Do surgical gloves protect staff during electrosurgical procedure? *Surgery* **110**: 892–5.

Chapter 6
Basic Laparoscopic Techniques
R.J.S. Hawthorn and K.F. Donaldson

Introduction

Basic techniques and approaches to laparoscopy are generally learned from one's seniors. Through time and working in different departments, various techniques and preferences are encountered. This chapter describes most of the popular techniques and explains the rationale behind them, with the emphasis being on safety. Consideration is also given to approaching safe operative and diagnostic laparoscopy using multiple ports of entry.

Patient selection

As in every branch of medicine, the importance of a good history, thorough examination and appropriate investigations cannot be emphasized strongly enough if one is to undertake the optimal procedure for the patient. In general, contraindications to a laparoscopic approach include severe cardiorespiratory compromise, gross obesity, and cardiac or respiratory disease that precludes general anaesthesia. Contraindications are listed below.

Contraindications to laparoscopic surgery

- Severe cardiac or respiratory disease
- Gross obesity
- Operator inexperience
- Lack of trained nursing staff
- Lack of suitable instruments or equipment

Once the decision to perform laparoscopy has been made, many units have simple guidelines as to which patients are suitable for day-case laparoscopy. Day-case surgery is appropriate for most women undergoing diagnostic laparoscopy and simple operative procedures such as sterilization.

Patient preparation

Patient counselling and preparation commences in the gynaecology clinic, particularly if complex operative laparoscopy is contemplated. In these circumstances, it should be stressed that a more rapid recovery to normal activities would be expected than with the

> # Key point
>
> The use of patient information booklets for laparoscopic surgery can pre-empt many common questions.

traditional open alternative. Other appropriate family members and the general practitioner should also be made aware that an early discharge and return to normal activities is likely. The use of information booklets for patients undergoing endoscopic surgery can help to pre-empt many of the common questions this surgery raises.

Assessment

Following admission, the results of any chest radiography and electrocardiography performed should be available. Other routine investigations are dependent on the procedure being performed. A full blood count for most patients is satisfactory and a 'grouped and retained' sample may be appropriate in some. With experience and audit of results, it may become apparent that having crossmatched blood available is not always required either, e.g. for laparoscopic hysterectomy. If pelvic examination suggests a possible mass, the results of abdominal and/or vaginal ultrasonography should be available as this may influence the laparoscopic approach.

The major preoperative considerations are listed below. Patients should be routinely fasted from midnight for morning procedures. Those scheduled for afternoon surgery may be allowed a light breakfast. Shaving of pubic hair is rarely indicated for simple diagnostic procedures or for minor operative procedures and should not be a matter of routine. Bowel preparation may be appropriate for some complex procedures, as the surgeon will prefer to operate in the pelvis of a patient whose large bowel is not distended and is therefore easier to manipulate. Anecdotal experience suggests that patients to whom bowel preparation is given experience less postoperative colicky and wind-type pain. In addition, the nurses in the ward and the patient

> # Preoperative considerations
>
> - Fasting
> - Shaving of pubic hair is rarely indicated
> - Bowel preparation
> - Antibiotic prophylaxis
> - Thromboembolism prophylaxis

herself will not then be concerned about bowel movements prior to discharge. Picolax (Ferring, Feltham, UK) given on the day before surgery is usually satisfactory. Information regarding the administration of Picolax can be obtained from the radiology department in most hospitals and sent to the patient if required.

Antibiotic prophylaxis should be considered, especially if laparoscopic hysterectomy or colposuspension is being undertaken. Similarly, thought should be given to reducing the possibility of deep vein thrombosis through the use of antiembolic stockings and subcutaneous heparin in procedures expected to last over an hour.

In planning the procedure the surgeon should take account of the likely time required to complete surgery. This involves detailed knowledge of any significant pathology, such as pelvic adhesions, large fibroids or previous surgery, that could substantially prolong the procedure. The surgeon's own experience will also be relevant, and theatre time should be planned accordingly.

Preparation and planning for the procedure should include ensuring that all equipment likely to be used is available close at hand. When equipment has been borrowed for a specific procedure it is important to check with the appropriate hospital department that indemnity has been obtained and that necessary electrical and compatibility checks have been carried out.

Consent

In counselling a patient for a specific procedure, it is generally accepted that complications occurring in more than 1% of cases should be mentioned to the patient. The exact complications discussed should be recorded in the patient's notes. A better method would be to have a specific consent form detailing the more frequent complications.

Most laparoscopic surgeons do not have experience of large personal series, but it would be reasonable to inform the patient of the operator's own experience of complications. Where the procedure is being undertaken for the first time, this should be explained to the patient and documented. The likely benefits and precautions being taken to ensure a successful outcome should be emphasized.

Where a visiting surgeon is the main operator, it is desirable that they be involved in the preoperative counselling and if possible in the postoperative care.

The risk of laparotomy for the individual procedure should be explained to all patients, preferably from the operator's own experience. This advice should be modified where the history and/or examination suggest that there are likely to be additional problems, particularly following previous pelvic surgery. However, in general terms, the risk of laparotomy is proportional to the complexity of the surgery being undertaken[1].

Position of the patient

The patient should be placed in the lithotomy position, but the hips should not be fully flexed as this severely impairs access for the surgeon. The feet should be held in lithotomy stirrups at an angle of about 30–45° to the horizontal to facilitate access. For longer procedures, Lloyd-Davis stirrups supporting the knees are to be preferred, as they give better support and limit the extent to which the patient slips up the table. A Trendelenburg tilt up to 30° may be required in some instances to displace the bowel from the pelvis. Shoulder supports may be required to maintain this position in some cases.

It is preferable if the patient's arms are placed by her side or across her chest, as the use of an arm board can limit access for the surgeon and assistant and make operating uncomfortable, particularly during long procedures.

The buttocks should be placed at the end of the operating table but not beyond as this puts strain on the lower back. If the buttocks are not at the end of the table, this significantly limits the uterine mobility that can be achieved.

Cleansing, catheterization and draping

The abdominal skin and perineum are usually cleansed with bactericidal and bacteriostatic solutions such as Savlon (ICI Pharmaceuticals, Macclesfield, UK) followed by chlorhexidine in spirit. The labia should be parted and the vagina cleansed. The bladder is then catheterized using an in/out catheter.

An indwelling Foley catheter may be used for longer procedures. Methylene blue may be instilled into the bladder where there is an additional risk of perforation, such as in laparoscopic hysterectomy following caesarean section and laparoscopic colposuspension. The simplest way to do this is to attach a 500 ml bag of normal saline containing the dye to the catheter. 200 ml of fluid should be removed before the bag is connected to the catheter to allow continuous bladder drainage throughout the procedure. Elevating the bag fills the bladder at any point should perforation be suspected.

Following catheterization a bimanual examination should be performed and an instrument placed in the uterus for manipulation. A Spackman cannula may be sufficient in some cases, but is not particularly efficient at mobilizing the body of the uterus. This may be achieved using a Hegar dilator or large curette. The most efficient but also the most expensive instrument is a Valtchev uterine manipulator (Conkin Surgical, Toronto, Canada; Figure 6.1).

The patient is draped using disposable drapes or standard sterile drapes. A specialized laparoscopic instrument holder such as a Hunt organizer (Figure 6.2) is useful where several instruments are likely to

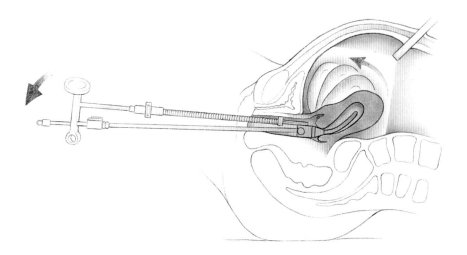

Figure 6.1 *Valtchev uterine manipulator.*

be needed. This disposable plastic organizer may be conveniently attached over the patient's leg after draping.

Establishment of safe pneumoperitoneum

Insertion of the Veress needle

Once the abdomen has been cleansed with antiseptic skin preparation the Veress needle should be connected to the carbon dioxide insufflator and patency tested at a low flow rate such as 1 l/min. Disposable or reusable Veress needles may be used. Where a reusable Veress needle is chosen, the spring-loaded barrel and not the needle should be grasped. The needle is usually inserted through or below the umbilicus or suprapubically following an initial skin incision (Figure 6.3). In the subumbilical approach the left hand grasps and elevates the abdominal wall. With the suprapubic approach the left hand is placed over the sacral promontory, and with the skin slightly stretched the needle is inserted, aiming towards the assistant's feet and thus into the pelvis below the bifurcation of the great vessels. In the obese patient, the umbilical approach using a long Veress needle should be employed, because the abdominal wall is thinnest at the umbilicus.

A new optical Veress needle (Storz, Tuttlingen, Germany) is now available but vision through such a small device is compromised.

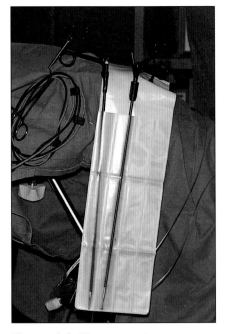

Figure 6.2 *Hunt organizer.*

Alternative insertion points

These approaches tend to be reserved for cases in which extensive bowel and/or omental adhesions in the midline are suspected; damage from the needle may thus be avoided.

Alternative sites are through the left upper quadrant (the ninth intercostal space), the pouch of Douglas or the fundus of the uterus. If the approach is through the pouch of Douglas a steep Trendelenburg

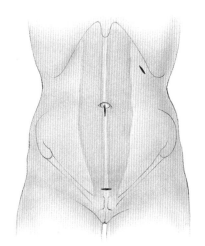

Figure 6.3 *Alternative insufflation sites.*

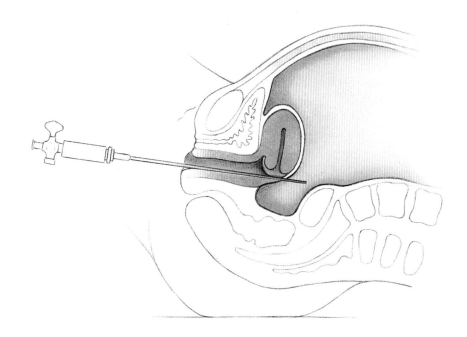

position is required to displace the small bowel. With the transfundal approach, it is important to sound the length of the uterine cavity before insertion of the needle.

Confirming the needle position

In experienced hands a double click may be heard and felt as the needle passes through the sheath and peritoneum. This is usually accompanied by free flow of the gas and a low intraperitoneal pressure recorded by the insufflator. Some authorities advocate moving the needle to ensure that it is freely mobile but this may tear small vessels, especially if the needle has passed through the small bowel mesentery.

Other tests include sniffing the end of the Veress needle and checking for a hiss as the abdominal wall is elevated, drawing air into the peritoneal cavity. A syringe filled with saline may be connected to the Veress needle. Correct placement is confirmed if fluid inserted into the peritoneum cannot be withdrawn.

Insufflating the peritoneum

Gas is then insufflated until a suitable pneumoperitoneum has been achieved, usually based on loss of liver dullness on percussion and visual appearance. The rate of carbon dioxide insufflation may be increased from 1 to 3 l/min, but flow rates much beyond this are not effectively achieved through the small-diameter Veress needle. With an electronic insufflator the maximum intra-abdominal pressure should be preset to 10 mmHg in the very thin patient. In the obese patient, a pressure of 12–15 mmHg may be used. If there is free gas flow the intra-abdominal pressure will rarely rise above 10 mmHg at 1 l/min.

Cannula selection and trocar insertion

Insertion of the primary trocar

The primary trocar is usually inserted after induction of the pneumoperitoneum; however, direct placement of the primary trocar into the peritoneum is described and may be the method of choice employed by some[2]. This approach should be used only by the experienced laparoscopist. The advantage of this approach is that extraperitoneal insufflation is avoided because the site is confirmed as intraperitoneal using the laparoscope before commencing insufflation.

The risk associated with the insertion of the primary trocar is perforation of a viscus or vascular damage. Guarded trocars (Figure 6.4) from Ethicon Endosurgical (Edinburgh, UK) and Auto Suture (Ascot, UK) are most valuable for the primary insertion but, in general, sharp pyramidal trocars are indicated for the initial puncture. A 10 mm cannula is most commonly used but a 12 mm cannula with a reducer should be considered if larger diameter operating instruments, such as the EndoGIA linear stapler (Auto Suture, Ascot, UK), are to be used from a midline approach. In this case, the laparoscope can be inserted via a lateral secondary port.

With the chosen trocar and cannula in the palm of the right hand, the operator should insert the trocar perpendicular to the skin with the index finger extended along the cannula to prevent uncontrolled entry. At the same time, the abdominal wall should be elevated and supported either with the left hand or by an assistant. The trocar should then be directed towards the pelvis and through the peritoneum.

Figure 6.4 *Guarded trocars. (Left) Endopath (courtesy of Ethicon, Edinburgh, UK) and (right) Versaport (courtesy of Auto Suture, Ascot, UK).*

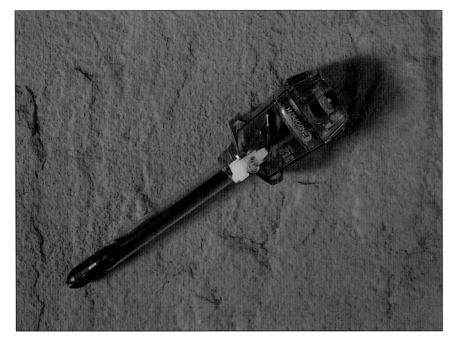

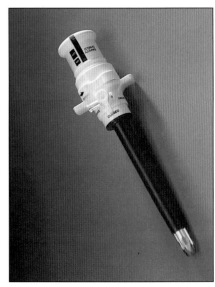

Hasson[3] described the technique of open laparoscopy (Figure 6.5). Using fine retractors and hooks a 10 mm skin incision in the umbilicus is deepened, the peritoneum opened under direct vision and the blunt-ended trocar and cannula inserted. Using fascial sutures the cannula is secured to skin and a movable cone placed to produce a tight seal. This technique is more commonly employed by general surgeons operating in the upper abdomen because a Trendelenburg position is not needed initially. Additionally, it has advantages in the obese and where adhesions in the region of the umbilicus are suspected.

An alternative approach in the presence of adhesions is to initially insert a 5 mm trocar and laparoscope in the left upper quadrant to determine an adhesion-free area around the umbilicus. Dissection of periumbilical adhesions can then be performed before insertion of the umbilical trocar under visual control.

Recently, optical trocars (Visiport, Auto Suture; Figure 6.6) have been developed in which the laparoscope is inserted into a blunt trocar and dissection through the layers of the abdominal wall is possible with some visual guidance. The value of this in the presence of dense adhesions is questionable, but it is certainly of value where extraperitoneal laparoscopy is being performed, e.g. in laparoscopic colposuspension.

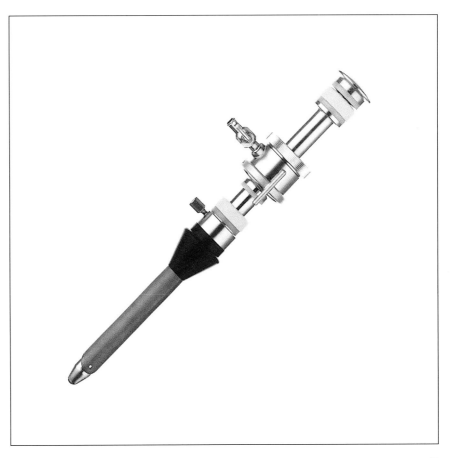

Figure 6.5 *Hasson open laparoscopy.*

Placement of secondary ports

In general, the placement of midline secondary ports poses little problem: cannulae are introduced under visual control through an appropriately sized skin incision. Where lateral ports are used, they should be placed lateral to the inferior epigastric vessels and rectus muscle. The site of lateral placement will be described under the appropriate procedure, but the technique should be standard.

The obliterated umbilical arteries should be easily visualized. The inferior epigastric vessels always lie laterally and may not be seen by simple transillumination other than in the very thin patient. The appropriate size skin incision should be made well lateral to these landmarks following Langer's skin cleavage lines. The handle of the scalpel may then be introduced through the incision at right-angles to the skin and the indentation in the peritoneum visualized through the laparoscope. The appropriate trocar is then introduced at a similar angle and the point of the trocar seen to penetrate the peritoneum before the trocar is angled towards the pelvis. It is negligent for secondary trocars to be introduced other than under visual guidance. Injury to bowel or to vessels is totally avoidable with these trocars.

It is important not to angle the trocar obliquely through the abdominal wall because the inferior epigastric vessels may be lacerated. In the obese patient, closure of these peritoneal incisions is much simpler if the skin incision overlies the peritoneal incision.

Types of cannula

Prior to insertion of additional ports, careful consideration must be given to the number and size of operating instruments likely to be used during the procedure. For linear staplers 12 mm ports are required, and these are also useful when relatively small amounts of tissue are to be removed intact through a port. The Steiner morcellator (Storz), for larger specimens, also requires the larger port size. Basic laparoscopic instruments, such as scissors and grasping and bipolar forceps, require only a 5 mm port. The newer ports with integral reducers will save time. In general, secondary ports with trumpet valves should be avoided as they can interfere with easy use of additional instruments. Usually two additional ports placed laterally are required but further midline access may be needed, particularly if laparoscopic suturing is required.

Plastic and metal cannula sleeves are available, some with integrated screw threads and others with separate collars to limit the penetration of the trocar into the peritoneum. The use of collars enlarges the wound size considerably. Sutures may be used to limit the mobility of the cannulae. Following the publication of the *Safety Action Bulletin* there has been a trend away from the use of plastic cannulae, but it is more important to avoid hybrid-type plastic cannulae with

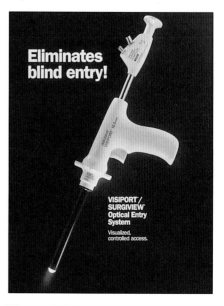

Figure 6.6 *Visiport optical trocar (courtesy of Auto Suture Company, Ascot, UK).*

metal collars and vice versa than to use all-metal cannulae. This is discussed further in Chapter 5 in relation to the use of diathermy at laparoscopic surgery.

Closure of portal wounds

There is growing evidence that all portal wounds greater than 10 mm should be effectively closed to reduce the incidence of Richter's and small-bowel hernias. Our experience indicates that both rectus sheath and peritoneal closure are also important. Various specialized devices are now available, including J-shaped and simple straight needles. In our experience, the most efficient closure has been achieved by reusable needles and a retriever (Maciol, Atlantic Healthcare, Johnstone, UK; Figure 6.7). This is also an effective method of dealing with bleeding from the abdominal wall.

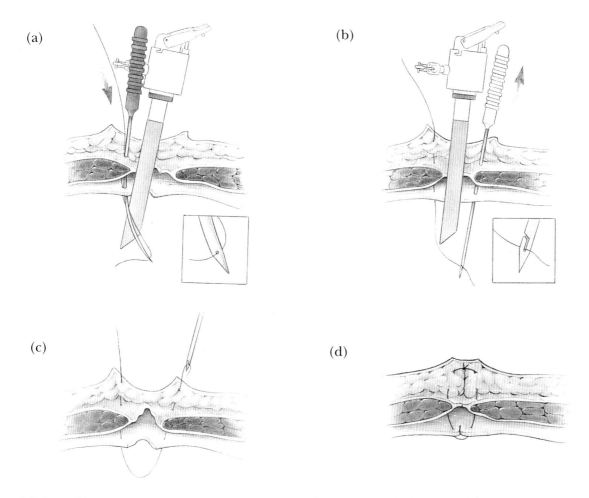

(a)   (b)

(c)   (d)

Figure 6.7 *Maciol laparoscopic suture needle set (redrawn with permission of Atlantic Healthcare, Johnstone, UK).*

Systematic approach to diagnostic laparoscopy

Following introduction of the laparoscope, a second port has to be introduced because it is impossible to perform adequate diagnostic laparoscopy using a single-puncture technique. If operative laparoscopy with multiple ports has to be performed, consideration must be given to structures that may be damaged during the course of the procedure. Most commonly, a 5 mm port is inserted suprapubically in the midline and an atraumatic grasping forceps used for manipulation. The practice of using a Veress needle as a probe is to be deprecated, as it not only damages the Veress needle but is also potentially dangerous, proving more traumatic to peritoneal tissue, and also affords a poorer view due to inadequate exposure.

Once the anatomy has been defined, the pelvis should be inspected in a systematic fashion, particularly for evidence of endometriosis. Detailed inspection usually commences with the assistant anteverting the uterus using the Spackman cannula or similar instrument to reveal the pouch of Douglas. Any peritoneal fluid should be aspirated via the Veress needle using a syringe to obtain a complete view. The uterosacral ligaments are examined for evidence of vesicles, powder burns or abnormal vascular patterns suggestive of endometriosis (Figure 6.8). These changes may become obvious only when the laparoscope is held close to the peritoneum, when magnification up to eight times is possible.

Each adnexa is then examined in turn, paying particular attention to the ovarian fossa and posterior surface of the ovary. This can only be achieved with the aid of an instrument inserted through the second port. The ovary may be flicked forward using a blunt probe, but a grasping forceps applied to the ovarian ligament is more effective.

The uterus is then retroverted, allowing the anterior surface of the uterus and the uterovesical fold of peritoneum to be inspected. Again, evidence of endometriosis is sought. In cases of pelvic pain, the appendix should also be examined together with the upper abdomen, in particular for the presence of perihepatic adhesions, the

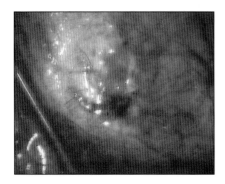 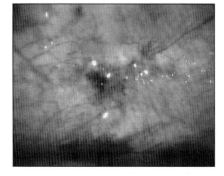 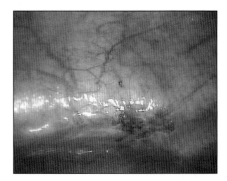

Figure 6.8 *Endometriosis.*

Fitz-Hugh–Curtis syndrome (Figure 6.9), an indication of previous chlamydial infection. If a diagnosis of pelvic varices is suspected, the patient should be tilted slightly head-up and, with the bowel displaced from the pelvis, the pelvic veins examined.

On completion of the procedure, the laparoscope and the second cannula are removed. The pneumoperitoneum is deflated through the umbilical cannula. Following removal of the umbilical cannula, both wounds are closed.

Record keeping

Detailed written notes of the findings are essential, but these can be considerably improved by the use of simple drawings. The availability of diagrams onto which findings can be recorded improves accuracy. With the newer technique of videolaparoscopy, the whole procedure can be recorded on videotape but, ultimately, this will cause problems with storage; a simple photograph produced through a video printer may be a suitable compromise, particularly if these are added to the case notes for future reference. A number of commercial systems are available using computers to capture images, which can be stored on electronic media. It is also possible to save images digitally. These may subsequently be enhanced for reproduction by systems that use optical computer disks (Litechnica, Heston, UK). Sony produce a similar single photograph-storing system on small computer disks at reasonable cost (Sony, Promavica system, Staines, UK). The Canon ION camera (Canon, Croydon, UK) allows direct input of the video

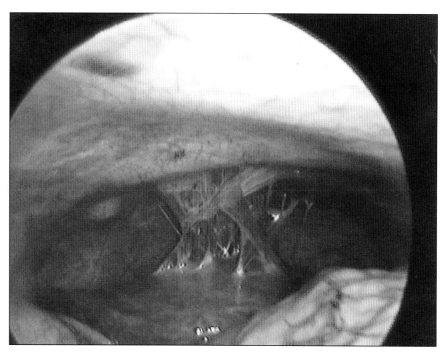

Figure 6.9 *Fitz-Hugh–Curtis syndrome.*

output, and images can be stored on a video floppy disk 40 mm in diameter for later retrieval.

The staging of endometriosis provides a good model for mapping the extent of disease[4]. The density and extent of adhesions and of tubal disease may be recorded in a similar detailed manner.

The detailed recording of results may be important when planning further surgery and assessing the outcome of medical treatment, and for explanation to patients and in medicolegal matters.

Summary

Almost all patients are suitable for laparoscopic surgery, the exceptions being those with severe degrees of cardiac or respiratory disease and with gross obesity. Laparoscopy should only be performed by surgeons trained in the basic principles of these procedures assisted by trained staff using suitable equipment. Patients require adequate assessment, counselling and information prior to consenting to a procedure which could lead unexpectedly to laparotomy. Bowel preparation should be performed prior to complex procedures. Care should be taken to position the patient, emptying the bladder, creating the pneumo–peritoneum and in placing the trocars. Findings at laparoscopy should be systematically made and recorded. Careful attention is required for closure of portal incisions 10 mm or larger to avoid herniation.

References

1   Bassil S, Nisolle M, Donnez J (1993) Complications of surgery in gynaecology. *Gynaecol Endosc* **2**: 199–209.
2. Phipps JH (1993) *Laparoscopic Hysterectomy and Oophorectomy: A Practical Manual and Colour Atlas.* Churchill Livingstone, Edinburgh, pp. 37–50.
3. Hasson HM (1978) Open laparoscopy *vs* closed laparoscopy: a comparison of complication rates. *Adv Planned Parenthood* **13**: 41–51.
4. American Fertility Society (1985) Revised Fertility Society classification of endometriosis. *Fertil Steril* **43**: 351.

Chapter 7

Laparoscopic Complications and How to Avoid Them

S.G. Harding and D.L. McMillan

Open laparoscopy

Trocar entry without prior establishment of
pneumoperitoneum
Miscellaneous methods

Major vascular injury

Perforation of the inferior epigastric vessels

Gastrointestinal injury

Trocar insertion injuries
Intraoperative bowel injury
Delayed bowel injury
Avoiding bowel injuries

Injury to the genitourinary system

Bladder injuries
Ureteric injuries
Anatomy
Preventing ureteric injury

Port closure and prevention of hernia

Adhesiolysis

Summary

Bibliography

Introduction

This chapter identifies the most commonly encountered complications of laparoscopic surgery and offers practical guidance on minimizing the risk of complications and on managing them when they arise.

Background

Laparoscopy, particularly in gynaecology, has been practised for many years although, until recently, this mode of access was chiefly confined to diagnostic and female sterilization procedures. Advances in technology have led to the development of minimally invasive surgical techniques.

The catalyst for these changes in laparoscopic surgery has been the silicon chip video camera, which has allowed us to enhance and magnify the image seen through the laparoscope so that precision is increased and tissue damage reduced. Video monitoring has expanded the role of assistants in endoscopic surgery, as they are able to view and participate in the operation along with the surgeon. Because of the technological improvements in instrumentation and the use of chip video cameras, it is now possible for at least 70% of all gynaecological operations to be performed laparoscopically.

DeCherney wrote, in 1985, 'The obituary for laparotomy for pelvic reconstructive surgery has been written; it is only its publication that remains ... In the 80's, a burgeoning of reconstructive surgery with the use of the endoscope will revolutionize gynaecological surgery'. Unfortunately, until recently, this has not been the view of the academic establishment in gynaecology, who regarded endoscopic surgery sceptically. This attitude, combined with an increased tendency among patients to seek out new treatments publicized in the media, led to the widespread introduction of laparoscopic surgical procedures without the prior scrutiny of prospective clinical trials, and with a number of surgeons undertaking procedures with inadequate training. A high rate of complications was, perhaps not surprisingly, encountered.

Patient expectations

The main advantages of endoscopic surgery compared with laparotomy are the lower patient morbidity and faster recovery time. However, the patient is more likely to consider the surgery to be minor and is therefore less tolerant of complications. Similarly, if a laparotomy is later found to be necessary, this causes more distress than if it had been performed initially. In addition, patient expectation of outcomes may be unrealistic. This is best demonstrated by the patient who believes that her endometriosis will finally be cured by the 'new laser treatment'.

The gynaecologist must ensure that the patient understands the nature and potential results of the procedures. This is no less important an issue than obtaining consent for other procedures, but potentially more of a problem because of high patient expectations. It would be prudent if, at least in the learning phase of endoscopic surgery, the gynaecologist operated endoscopically only on patients who would otherwise benefit from conventional surgery, and ensured that the patient was aware of this. In this case, proceeding to an unexpected laparotomy is less likely to be seen as an indication of failure of care.

Medicolegal implications of video monitoring

This presents a new medicolegal issue which has not been completely addressed. Consent must be obtained if recorded procedures are to be used for lectures or demonstrations. In other circumstances, recording of the procedure might be considered to be an extension of the patient's medical record, and might be required as evidence in the event of litigation. Videotapes should be stored as carefully as other medical records, so that they are available for review if required.

Preoperative examination

When setting out to perform laparoscopic surgery, it is essential to acquire as much information as possible about the condition to be treated, because this will dictate, firstly, whether the surgeon is sufficiently skilled and trained to perform the operation and, secondly, the likely length of time that the procedure will take. Ultrasonography, particularly transvaginal ultrasonography, is extremely useful in the diagnosis of ovarian cysts, benign and malignant tumours, and uterine abnormalities. The presence of fibroids can be detected and their exact size, number and location determined.

Complications associated with pneumoperitoneum

The majority of complications in laparoscopic surgery occur at the time of abdominal entry. Surgeons performing laparoscopic techniques should have the ability to recognize and deal with any complications that might arise. All patients should be assessed before surgery, and any problems that might arise with respect to the establishment of a pneumoperitoneum should be considered along with measures to avoid them.

Site selection

The site of the Veress needle insertion is dictated by the individual patient's characteristics, not necessarily by the surgeon's preference for a particular site. Scars from previous abdominal surgery may make the use of the traditional intraumbilical insertion point hazardous, and alternative sites of entry may need to be selected (Figure 7.1).

One of the sites associated with the lowest incidence of morbidity is the suprapubic site. The Veress needle is inserted vertically in the midline and passed through the deep fascia and the peritoneum until it touches the uterus, which is manipulated vaginally. This method is considered to be suitable for surgeons who are commencing their training in laparoscopy, as the complication rate is low. The main contraindication to this method is pregnancy, as the fundus of the soft pregnant uterus is difficult to palpate. If the Veress needle punctures the pregnant uterus, carbon dioxide may enter the venous circulation through the venous sinuses, and fatal carbon dioxide embolism can ensue. This can be considered a safe technique for insertion only if pregnancy is excluded.

Most experienced surgeons agree that the lower edge of the umbilical depression is the area of choice. At this point, the peritoneum joins the umbilical plate, thus considerably reducing the distance the Veress needle needs to traverse through the peritoneal fat (Figure 7.2). The incision should only be large enough to allow the insertion of the Veress needle in the first instance in case a pneumoperitoneum is not established and alternative sites of insertion need to be considered.

Veress needle insertion

Initially the patency and spring mechanism of the Veress needle should be checked. Insertion of the Veress needle should be made through the deepest part of the umbilicus, because at this point the abdominal wall is thin and the peritoneum is at the closest point to the skin. The area of the lower abdomen just above the symphysis pubis is grasped by the surgeon's left hand and elevated upward and cephalad at a 45° angle to the horizontal. This slightly elevates the umbilicus,

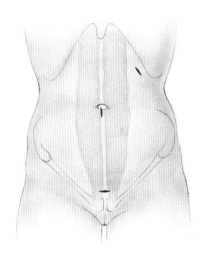

Figure 7.1 *Sites for Veress needle insertion. The needle may also be inserted through the posterior vaginal fornix.*

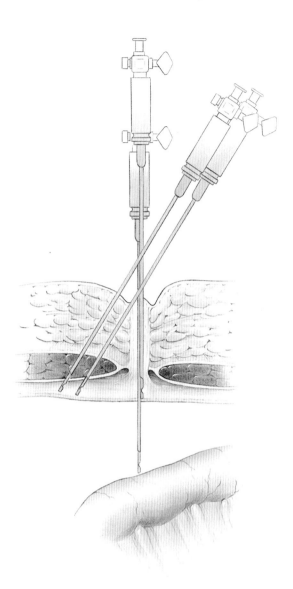

Figure 7.2 *Differences in the depth of the anterior wall at the level of the umbilicus.*

placing its underlying peritoneum on a stretch in a plane roughly perpendicular to the axis of the true pelvis. The Veress needle is then grasped in the surgeon's right hand with the upper barrel between the thumb and index finger, with the fourth finger of the right hand resting on the shaft of the needle guarding against the needle being inserted too far into the peritoneal cavity (Figure 7.3).

The Veress needle can then be inserted at right-angles to the skin (45° caudad off the vertical) straight into the axis of the true pelvis.

Throughout the insertion of the Veress needle the patient should be kept horizontal, because only the horizontal plane provides reference to the underlying anatomy. The practice of tilting the patient in a Trendelenburg position before the establishment of a pneumoperitoneum is, in our opinion, unsafe practice (Figure 7.4).

Figure 7.3 *Veress needle insertion, with the fourth finger of the right hand on the shaft of the needle.*

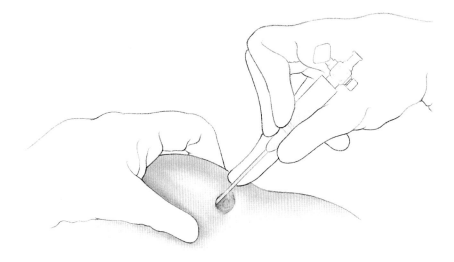

Figure 7.4 *Alteration of anatomy due to the Trendelenburg position.*

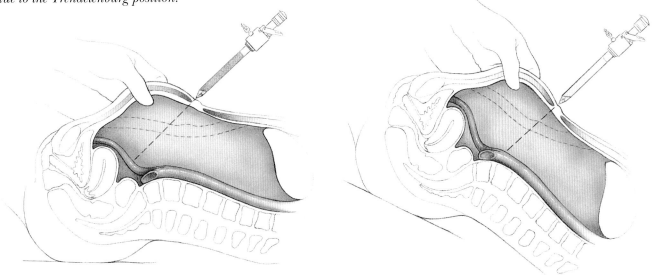

Confirmation of peritoneal entry

After the insertion of the Veress needle, there are several available tests to ensure that the tip of the Veress needle is indeed within the peritoneal cavity. Several Veress needles are now available with hollow chambers containing a small ball above the spring mechanism. These devices make an audible click on piercing the rectus sheath and then again on entering the peritoneum which, although not an absolute test of peritoneal entry, is a useful addition to the tests outlined below.

Syringe test

A 10 ml syringe is filled with saline and attached to the Veress needle. 5 ml are then injected and the plunger is withdrawn. No aspirate should be obtained if the needle is in the peritoneal cavity as the fluid will have dispersed between loops of bowel (Figure 7.5a). If the needle lies in the abdominal wall (Figure 7.5b) clear fluid will be withdrawn. If, however, the aspirate is stained red or brown, perforation of bowel or blood vessel has occurred and the surgeon must decide how best to proceed with the operation.

If the fluid is clear the plunger is removed from the syringe and the residual saline is allowed to flow into the peritoneal cavity (Figure 7.5c). If the needle is supraperitoneal the fluid may dissipate itself into the peritoneal fat but its flow will be much slower. Elevation of the lower abdominal wall creating negation pressure should lead to a much faster flow if the needle is correctly situated.

Swinging needle test

The needle is swung in an arc and the surgeon determines whether the needle tip is swinging in a counter arc with the pivot point at the rectus fascia midway down the needle. If the needle is swinging with its pivot point at its tip, the needle is probably above the peritoneum and should be reinserted more deeply (Figure 7.6). One should obviously bear in mind that the tip of the Veress needle cannot be visualized during this procedure, and moving it without due care may damage the abdominal viscera. For this reason the test is eschewed by many experienced surgeons.

Direct Veress needle insertion with optical catheter

The last blind entry! Recently, optical catheters have been designed which will fit inside a Veress needle and allow the surgeon to directly visualize entry into the abdominal cavity.

Insufflation

Once the surgeon is satisfied that the Veress needle is in the peritoneal space, the gas flow is attached and insufflation is commenced, initially at no more than 1 l/min, ensuring that intra-abdominal pressure does not exceed 15 mmHg. If slight elevations of the intra-abdominal pressure coincide with the patient's expiration, the needle is probably in the peritoneal space.

Percussion of the right hypochondrium should demonstrate the loss of liver dullness when approximately 400 ml of gas has entered the peritoneal cavity. (This is also approximately the amount of carbon dioxide that can enter the vascular system without compromising the patient, if a blood vessel is inadvertently punctured with the Veress needle.) Inspection of the gradual abdominal distension should show the abdomen filling uniformly; if the needle is in the supraperitoneal space, the lower abdomen will distend without a concomitant distension of the upper abdomen.

High pressure

The opening at the tip of the Veress needle is always on the same side as the valve lever, which should be directed downwards to avoid the

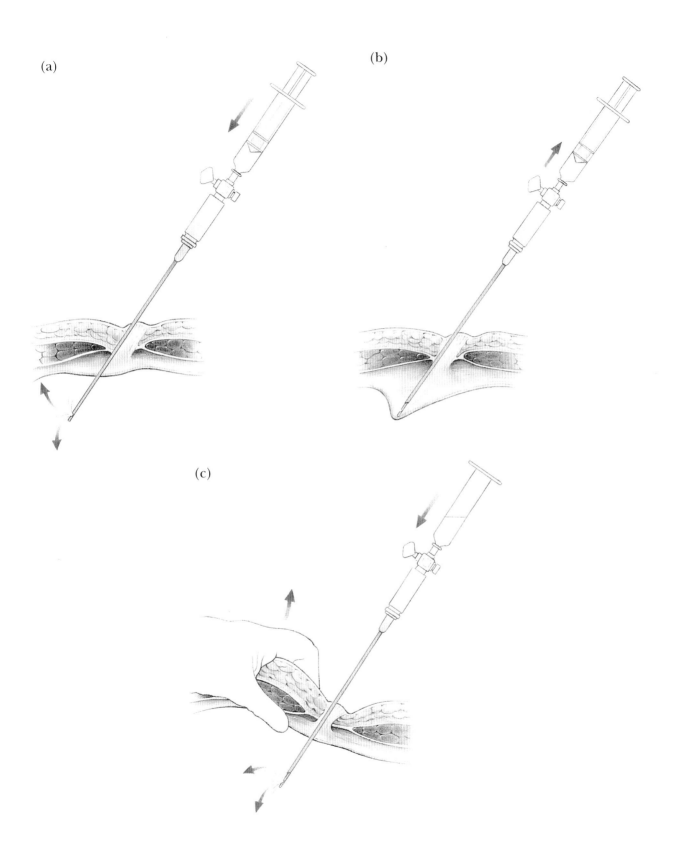

(a)

(b)

(c)

Figure 7.5 *Syringe test.*

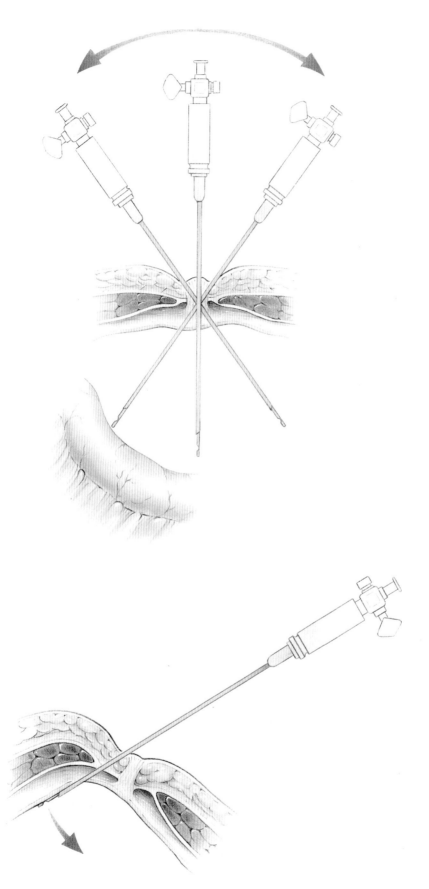

Figure 7.6 *The swinging needle test.*

Figure 7.7 *The Veress needle positioned against the peritoneum.*

peritoneum obstructing the opening (Figure 7.7). High insufflation pressures may also be caused by tissue blocking the needle tip. Flushing with 5 ml of saline should clear this problem.

Erratic pressure readings can be caused by residual water in the insufflation tubing after rinsing, and will clear in due course. If irregular high pressures persist, a supraperitoneal insertion should be suspected. In this case, insufflation should be discontinued, the pocket of gas evacuated, and a second effort made at reaching the peritoneum.

Repeated insertion attempts

Repeated unsuccessful attempts to enter the peritoneal cavity can result in the preperitoneal tissue being dissected away from the peritoneum. In such circumstances, an alternative site of entry needs to be considered. Entry via an incision in the left hypochondrium would be the chosen alternative (1 cm lateral to the costochondral junction to avoid the superior epigastric vessels). This site is preferred as there are unlikely to be adhesions from previous intra-abdominal inflammation or surgery (e.g. cholecystitis or diverticular disease) and this point of entry avoids the dissected peritoneum in the lower abdomen. Alternative insertions can be made through the posterior fornix of the vagina or through the upper left margin of the umbilicus (to avoid ligamentum teres). However, beware of the abdominal aorta lying directly underneath.

When the peritoneum is positively reached after this process, it is advisable to inflate the abdomen beyond the normal 15 mmHg. This elevated intra-abdominal pressure will hold the dissected peritoneum against the preperitoneal fat and allow an easier insertion of the first trocar. During this time, the anaesthetist should be kept fully informed so that any respiratory difficulties caused by diaphragmatic pressure can be anticipated.

Failed entry

Because laparoscopy tends to be on the whole an elective procedure, we should allow ourselves three attempts before considering abandoning the procedure. At this point, the patient's abdominal wall has been transversed repeatedly and the surgeon will be becoming increasingly concerned. At this juncture, it is better to adjourn rather than compromise the patient's physical wellbeing. It may be prudent to call upon an experienced colleague, if one is easily available, as another surgeon coming fresh to the situation may be more successful. Open laparoscopy or minilaparotomy may be an alternative, although most elective procedures can be postponed to another day.

Trocar insertion

Trocar insertion is the most hazardous part of the procedure. The principles involved are similar to those outlined previously relating to the insertion of the Veress needle. Trocars need to be extremely sharp to facilitate easy and unforced entry to the abdominal cavity. This, and the fact that the initial trocar is generally inserted blind, carries a risk of visceral trauma.

If there are suspected adhesions at the proposed site of entry of the trocar, the peritoneal space below the umbilicus can be explored with a needle. If gas cannot be aspirated freely after probing in several directions, adhesions of bowel or omentum should be suspected. The surgeon should then either consider an alternative site for trocar entry or perform an open laparoscopy.

The primary objective is to keep the trocar point as far away from the pelvic vessels as possible. This is achieved either by elevating the lower abdominal wall with the left hand or by pressing the left forearm against the patient's upper abdomen, forcing most of the intra-abdominal gas into the lower abdomen. Both of these techniques ensure that the distance between the trocar point and the major vessels is at its maximum.

The use of trocars that automatically guard their point when they meet no resistance should be encouraged, although there have been cases of visceral injury with these disposable trocars.

A vertical incision is made from the deepest point of the umbilicus in an outward direction, the size of which depends on the laparoscope being used. The trocar should be aimed at the uterus and kept vertically in the midline as deviation to the left or right of the midline can result in damage to the pelvic vessels. When teaching laparoscopic techniques, it is useful to observe trainees from the foot of the operating table to ensure that they are adhering to the midline.

Some surgeons favour insertion through a zig-zag path to avoid hernia formation. However, extreme caution must be exercised since undue force applied during this technique may lead to trauma to the great vessels of the posterior wall of the abdomen.

As the trocar passes through the abdominal wall and enters the peritoneal cavity, the surgeon should twice feel a distinct loss of resistance to the passage of the trocar, the second indicating that the trocar has successfully breached the peritoneum. At this point, the trocar should be held under a slight forward pressure and the trocar sleeve advanced on its own for about 5 cm or, in obese women, until the trumpet valve touches the skin. This ensures that the sleeve is well

Safety point

The patient should be kept horizontal during trocar insertion to maintain the surgeon's orientation to the underlying anatomy (Figure 7.4).

Figure 7.8 Zig-zag trocar insertion.

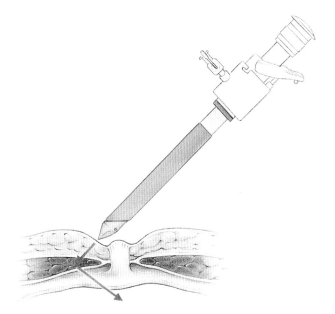

within the peritoneal cavity and will not be inadvertently withdrawn above the peritoneum when the trocar is removed.

When the trocar is withdrawn, the trumpet valve is briefly kept open and the gush of gas confirms entry into the peritoneum.

A laparoscope that has been warmed (to prevent fogging) is then inserted past the trumpet valve but kept within the sleeve.

Laparoscopic inspection (Figure 7.9) should first be directed downwards to observe any dripping of blood along the side of the

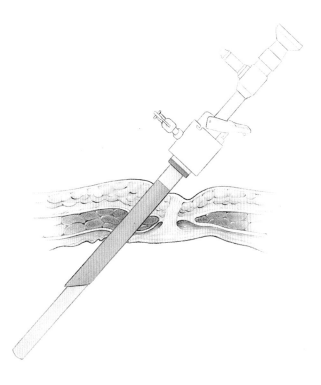

Figure 7.9 *Initial laparoscopic inspection.*

sleeve, which suggests vessel damage at the insertion point. The laparoscope is then extended beyond the end of the sleeve, allowing observation of the viscera directly below the trocar site. If adhesions are identified, the laparoscope should be advanced past them carefully and into the abdominal cavity; it is then prudent to view the first portal of entry from another site to ensure that there is no bowel involved in the adhesions. If, after these manoeuvres, the laparoscope is not in the abdominal cavity, the procedure should be abandoned. A laparotomy should be contemplated if there is any suspicion of damage to intra-abdominal organs.

After careful inspection of the upper abdomen, the patient is placed in a modified Trendelenburg position (25°) to facilitate the moving of bowel away from the pelvis. At this stage, any additional trocar insertion points need to be considered and the plan of surgery established. The most usual points for insertion are shown below in Figure 7.10.

The size of the skin incision should be checked using the trocar sleeve to ensure that undue force is not used to push the trocar past too small an incision. Keeping the forefinger extended on the sleeve will prevent the trocar from being inserted too deeply.

The techniques outlined above are our preferred methods of laparoscopic surgery. These have been developed from personal experience and observation of the methods employed by several of the leading exponents of operative laparoscopy. There are many alternatives to the described techniques which in experienced hands give excellent results. They can, however, be hazardous if performed by inexperienced operators. The methods which we have outlined will in our opinion result in safe practice and are easy to teach to trainees.

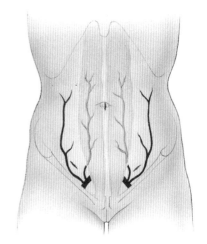

Figure 7.10 Trocar insertion sites.

Open laparoscopy

A 2–3 cm skin incision is made subumbilically in a vertical plane. Small Deaver retractors are used to expose the underlying fascial planes to allow dissection onto the peritoneum. Two strong sutures are placed on the edges of the rectus sheath, and are used for elevation of the abdominal wall to facilitate entry into the peritoneal cavity. The peritoneum is incised and a purse-string suture is inserted through which a cannula without its trocar is passed into the peritoneal cavity. The purse-string is then tightened to make a seal. Gas is insufflated and the laparoscopy proceeds as normal. Alternatively, a Hasson trocar with obturator may be used to ensure a good seal at the entry site. On completion of the operation, the rectus sheath can be closed by tying the elevating sutures. Closure of the peritoneum is not essential.

This method was first described by Harrith Hasson in 1974 and used to minimize the risk of large vessel injury at the time of trocar insertion. It is particularly useful when intra-abdominal adhesions are suspected or following a failed insertion of the Veress needle.

Trocar entry without prior establishment of pneumoperitoneum

Although this technique flies in the face of convention, with proper patient selection it can reduce operating time and therefore anaesthesia time in busy units. It is used with good effect in sterilization units in the Third World.

The abdominal wall is elevated, as described previously, and the trocar inserted without the establishment of a pneumoperitoneum. The guidelines outlined previously must be rigidly observed with particular attention paid to the underlying anatomy, adequate skin incision at the trocar site and sharp instrumentation. After the trocar has entered the peritoneal cavity, air is allowed to enter the abdomen by gently elevating the cannula. The laparoscope is inserted into the cannula to view its end to ensure that it is in the peritoneal cavity. Omentum and bowel will be seen to move freely under the cannula, whereas supraperitoneal fat will not. After this has been established, the cavity can be insufflated and inspected, saving time on blind insufflation and testing. This technique is particularly appropriate in sterilization procedures where previous pregnancy has distended the abdominal walls, making them thinner and easier to elevate for trocar insertion. This technique should not be used where there has been previous abdominal surgery that could have led to adhesion formation.

Miscellaneous methods

The left hypochondrial entry (Palmer's point, 3 cm inferior to the left costal margin in the midclavicular line) is often useful in patients with distended paraumbilical veins, as seen with portal hypertension in liver disease.

Towel clips can be used to elevate the abdominal wall, although this requires an additional pair of hands.

Some practitioners ask the patient, under local anaesthesia, to bear down during trocar entry. The effect of this is to elevate the abdomen above the peritoneum and create a rigid structure through which the trocar can be inserted. This method is of particular interest to those now performing diagnostic laparoscopy under local anaesthesia using the newer laparoscopes, which are only 3.5 mm in diameter. With improved optics and the use of anaesthetic gases for insufflation, the possibility of operative laparoscopy under local anaesthetic will become a reality in the very near future.

Major vascular injury

In published reports, the risk of major vessel trauma during laparoscopy is 1 in 1000 cases; from this one can deduce that most

> # Key point
>
> The risk of major vessel trauma during laparoscopy is 1 in 1000.

gynaecologists will experience at least one of these potentially fatal incidents during their career. This accepted, however, the vast majority of laparoscopic major vessel injuries are preventable.

Every vessel within reach of the laparoscopic surgeon is at risk of damage. Trauma to the epigastric vessels, the mesenteric vessels, the inferior vena cava, abdominal aorta and iliac vessels have all been reported, with two-thirds of these injuries associated with Veress needle insertion. As long as the surgeon does not stray laterally from the midline with the Veress needle or primary trocar, the external or internal iliac vessels will not be at risk. The middle sacral artery, however, is at risk in the midline from too vigorous insertion of the Veress needle.

If blood is expelled through the Veress needle or primary cannula, major vessel injury should be suspected and an immediate laparotomy performed. Central venous access should be obtained and blood crossmatched.

A sudden drop in the patient's blood pressure when it is not associated with bradycardia, and is therefore unlikely to be a vasovagal response, should be considered to be due to a vascular accident until proved otherwise.

If free blood is visible in the peritoneal cavity when the laparoscope is inserted, the abdominal contents must be carefully inspected, particularly the omental and mesenteric vessels. The bowel must be moved to inspect the posterior peritoneum. Any obvious haemorrhage or haematoma collection in this area necessitates immediate laparotomy and compression of the bleeding vessel until assistance is available from a vascular surgeon.

Perforation of the inferior epigastric vessels

This is one of the most frequent laparoscopic complications: every laparoscopic surgeon will encounter one of these bleeding vessels from time to time, but it is much more likely in the following circumstances.

In the obese patient it is difficult to transilluminate these vessels, and the increased depth of the fatty layer makes perpendicular insertion of secondary trocars difficult. This is a particular problem with suprapubic trocars which can inadvertently be misdirected laterally and damage these vessels.

Previous abdominal surgery, particularly through low transverse abdominal incisions, often obscures the course of these vessels, putting them at greater risk of perforation.

Operations that require multiple secondary ports, or poor initial planning of where the ports should be located leading to reinsertion of secondary trocars, will place the inferior epigastric vessels at greater risk. This is particularly so if the larger, 10–11 mm, trocars are used. Laparoscopic surgeons must take great care with the insertion of every trocar: damage to the inferior epigastric artery will produce retroperitoneal or intraperitoneal bleeding and, to the superficial epigastric, intramuscular or subcutaneous bleeding. These vessels cannot be transilluminated except in very thin patients and need to be visualized from within the peritoneal cavity. Their origin can be traced from the emergence of the round ligament from the deep inguinal ring along the lateral margin of the rectus muscle. The obliterated umbilical ligaments are nearly always identifiable as they course from the umbilicus along the anterior abdominal wall, and provide a useful landmark as this ligament rarely lies outside the lateral edge of the rectus muscle. Placement of secondary trocars well lateral to the edge of the rectus muscle should, therefore, avoid injury to the inferior and superficial epigastric vessels (Figure 7.11).

It is important to remember that the location of the secondary port is irrelevant if the trocar is not inserted perpendicular to the fascia. Often, in obese patients, it is difficult to keep the trocar at 90° to the fascia, and this will place the inferior epigastric vessels at a greater risk of perforation.

Should these precautions fail to prevent bleeding at the secondary port, rotating the cannula through 360° will often produce

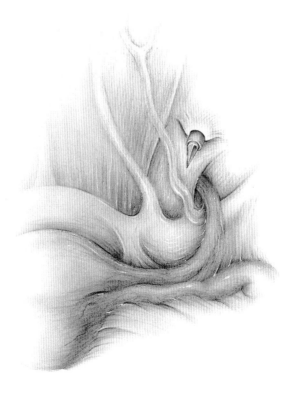

Figure 7.11 *Placement of secondary trocars.*

sufficient vessel tamponade to arrest the haemorrhage. If the bleeding continues, the cannula should be left *in situ* and on no account removed. Long bipolar forceps can be used to desiccate the vessels, both proximally and distally to the port. If a haematoma is present, it should be opened and evacuated using a suction/irrigation system until a clear effluent is obtained.

Another useful method of tamponading these vessels is to pass a Foley catheter through the offending cannula into the peritoneal cavity, inflate the balloon and withdraw the cannula until the catheter balloon tamponades the bleeding skin vessel. Further pressure can be exerted by securing a pad of swabs between the surface of the abdominal wall and an artery forceps gripping the Foley catheter.

Bleeding from vessels deep in the anterior abdominal wall is best controlled by inserting large hand-held curved needles through the whole thickness of the abdominal wall. The intra-abdominal course of this suture can be viewed laparoscopically, and these sutures should be placed cephalad and caudad to the cannula.

Lastly, it is important to remember that, although haemorrhage from the arterial supply to the anterior abdominal wall will be obvious as soon as the vessel is punctured, venous haemorrhage may be tamponaded by the pressure of the intraperitoneal gas and not reveal itself until this is released at the completion of the operation. It is extremely important to view all secondary ports after their cannulae are removed and the intraperitoneal gas has been released, to observe any sign of haemorrhage. Failure to do this after the completion of every laparoscopic procedure will eventually result in a collapsed patient in the recovery room.

Gastrointestinal injury

Trocar insertion injuries

Injury to the gastrointestinal tract occurs in 1.6–1.8 per 1000 laparoscopic procedures, with only 60% of these injuries being noted at the time of surgery. The most common time for injury to the gastrointestinal tract to occur is during the insertion of the Veress needle or primary trocar. This may be due to careless technique or immobilization of the bowel by adhesions (Figure 7.12). Patients who are particularly prone to bowel adhesions to the anterior abdominal wall are those with a history of multiple laparotomies (particularly with longitudinal scars), prior ruptured appendix or diverticulum, overdistended bowel or disseminated carcinoma.

In the absence of adhesions or other predisposing conditions the use of excessive force when inserting the primary trocar reduces the distance of the trocar from the underlying bowel, placing it at greater risk of damage. This is also true of an inadequate pneumoperitoneum.

Figure 7.12 *Bowel may be adherent to the anterior abdominal wall increasing the risk of injury.*

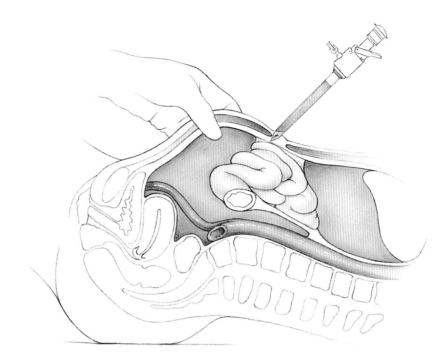

Factors such as too small an umbilical incision, scar tissue from a previous laparoscopy or other surgical procedure and a dull trocar lead to excessive force being used during the insertion of the primary trocar. Trocar insertion may also be difficult in very thin or obese patients.

Perforation of the bowel by the Veress needle is undoubtedly more common than is recognized, but is not a serious problem unless tearing of the bowel has occurred (which is avoided as long as the Veress needle is not blindly waved about in the peritoneal cavity after its insertion). If it is suspected by the characteristic faeculent smell on withdrawal of the Veress needle, the laparoscopy should proceed and the bowel below the insertion site should be inspected for any tears. As long as none are apparent, the patient can be managed expectantly.

Injury with the primary trocar is a far more major problem. It is imperative that this is diagnosed at the time of the laparoscopy, otherwise potentially fatal peritonitis will ensue. This most commonly arises when a loop of bowel (usually the transverse colon) is adherent to the anterior abdominal wall. The primary trocar may then skewer

Key point

Injury to the gastrointestinal tract occurs in 1.6–1.8 per 1000 laparoscopic procedures.

the bowel, passing through its full thickness, and this may go completely unnoticed by the surgeon. It is extremely important that the surgeon observes the site with the laparoscope within the cannula as it is removed, to avoid missing this particular injury.

If a trocar is inadvertently inserted into adhesions or bowel, the trocar should be removed allowing the cannula to remain in place so that if bowel has been perforated the site of perforation can be identified. It has been well described that, when the trocar and cannula have been withdrawn after a suspected perforation, it may be very difficult to locate the site of the perforation.

Intraoperative bowel injury

Bowel injury occurs most commonly during dissection of the rectosigmoid colon, particularly in patients with extensive cul de sac disease from endometriosis. Recognizing this type of injury can often be difficult. If damage is suspected but not evident laparoscopically, a Foley catheter can be passed into the rectum, its balloon inflated to 30 ml and Betadine (Napp Laboratories, Cambridge, UK) solution instilled above the balloon; any leakage through a full-thickness injury will then be demonstrated. Defects involving the full thickness of the bowel will need to be repaired by an experienced surgeon either by laparoscopy or by laparotomy. Superficial defects to the serosal layer can be managed expectantly with careful postoperative observation.

Small superficial thermal injuries to the bowel noticed during surgery can be treated prophylactically with a laparoscopically placed purse-string suture. This should be placed beyond the thermally affected tissue.

Delayed bowel injury

Delayed diagnosis of bowel injury may arise because the injury was not detected at the time of surgery or because the bowel sustained thermal damage that led to a delayed necrosis and subsequent perforation. In traumatic perforation the symptoms and signs will present within 24–48 h of surgery. Injuries due to thermal damage may not present for 10 days. These patients will present with fever, rigors and abdominal pain. The physical signs may vary from a rigid abdomen to only localized tenderness, depending on the extent of faecal contamination of the peritoneal cavity. Plain abdominal radiographs are often unhelpful because of residual carbon dioxide within the abdominal cavity mimicking free air from a perforated viscus, and barium contrast studies are contraindicated in a patient suspected of bowel perforation. It is therefore imperative that any patient with an acute abdomen following laparoscopic surgery undergoes immediate laparotomy with surgical exploration of the abdominal cavity, including the intestinal tract, to identify the cause.

Avoiding bowel injuries

Because bowel injury is generally associated with poor technique or bowel adhesions and distension, knowledge of these predisposing factors facilitates avoiding these complications.

The surgeon's standard trocar insertion technique should be safe (as outlined previously in this chapter) and not deviated from without good cause. The trocar should be sharp to facilitate easy penetration of the muscle and fascia. Disposable trocars offer a sharp tip and a spring-loaded safety shield, and should, theoretically, be safer. However, to the uninitiated, this ease of abdominal insertion may itself give rise to visceral trauma.

It is important to establish an adequate pneumoperitoneum before trocar insertion to maximize the distance between the abdominal wall and the underlying viscera, and all but the primary trocar should be inserted under direct vision.

The primary trocar should be inserted with the patient in the horizontal position, as a premature Trendelenburg position does nothing to avoid bowel injuries, particularly if adhesions are present, and significantly alters the surgeon's perception of the underlying anatomy.

Bowel distension secondary to obstruction is a relative contraindication. However, bowel distension can be iatrogenic, caused by the intraluminal placement of the Veress needle. Once the apparent pneumoperitoneum is created and the Veress needle is removed, the distended bowel is an easy target for the primary trocar. In the main, this type of complication can be avoided if the surgeon uses the simple techniques for confirmation of peritoneal entry outlined earlier in this chapter.

Injury to the genitourinary system

Bladder injuries

The urinary bladder is particularly prone to injury during the insertion of a low midline secondary trocar, bladder dissection from the anterior wall of the uterus during hysterectomy, and colposuspension when the patient has previously had a hysterectomy. The insufflation of an indwelling urinary catheter bag is often the first

---

Safety point

If the surgeon is suspicious of adhesions around the umbilicus due to previous surgery, alternative sites for insertion of the Veress needle or an open laparoscopy should be considered.

indication of this problem, as is the failure of the bladder to fill during a prolonged procedure. As with other complications, the cardinal step in the management of this problem is early recognition. If a perforation is found, a Foley's catheter should be placed in the bladder for 5–7 days and prophylactic antibiotics administered. The defect may be closed laparoscopically in two layers or, if small (<5 mm), free drainage of the bladder will suffice.

Ureteric injuries

It is well documented that the ureter is involved in complications during open surgery. It is now becoming evident that the ureter is also susceptible to injury during laparoscopic surgery, particularly in the procedures listed below.

Laparoscopic procedures in which the ureter may be damaged

- Laparoscopic uterine nerve ablation
- Laparoscopic hysterectomy (when the uterine artery is secured laparoscopically)
- Oophorectomy for a residual ovary following previous hysterectomy
- Surgery in patients with America Fertility Society stage IV endometriosis

---

Anatomy

Knowledge of the course of the pelvic ureter is mandatory for all gynaecological surgeons, and it should be remembered that the ureter's anatomical relations can alter dramatically with the various disease processes that are encountered in the gynaecological patient – particularly endometriosis.

The ureter enters the pelvis at the pelvic brim, crossing over the common iliac artery and vein. It then courses caudad, crossing under the uterine artery, entering the cardinal ligament, coming anteriorly and medially to enter the trigone of the bladder. At the level of the cervix, the ureter is 1–1.5 cm lateral to the uterosacral ligament (Figure 7.13).

The surgeon will most often encounter the ureter at the level of infundibulopelvic ligament (oophorectomy), of the uterine artery (laparoscopic hysterectomy) or of the cervix (laparoscopic uterine nerve ablation (LUNA)) (Figure 7.14).

Figure 7.13 *The ureter may lie close to the lateral border of the uterosacral ligaments and is particularly vulnerable during LUNA procedures.*

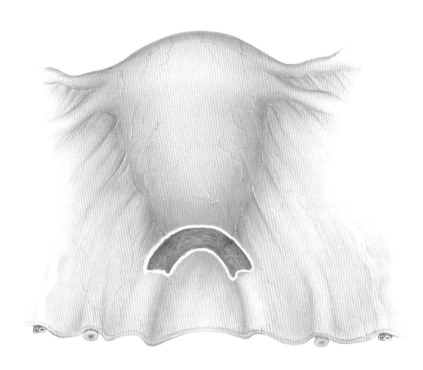

Figure 7.14 *Sites of ureteric injury: (a) at the pelvic brim, (b) where the ureter crosses under the uterine artery, (c) near the anterior fornix of the vagina (d) at the lateral pelvic sidewall, (e) in the intramural portion of the bladder.*

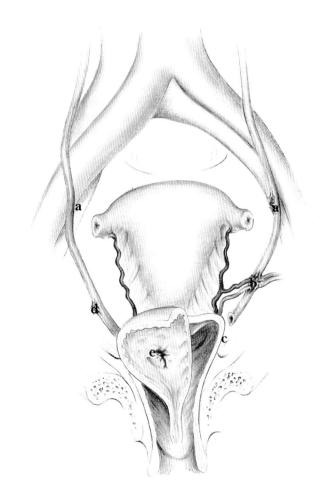

Preventing ureteric injury

There are some relatively simple methods that can be employed to prevent injury during the operations in which the ureter is most at risk.

During LUNA procedures the ureter should be identified as it approaches the uterosacral ligament, and a peritoneal incision made between the ureter and the ligament. The ureter can then be mobilized laterally with either blunt or hydrodissection. There can be no indication for performing a repeat LUNA procedure, as the scarring from the previous surgery will place the ureter at great risk of injury and is extremely unlikely to relieve the patient's symptoms if the first procedure failed to do so.

In laparoscopic hysterectomy, unless the ureter has been identified by either dissection or the insertion of ureteric stents, it is extremely vulnerable as it passes beneath the uterine artery. This is particularly so when endoscopic stapling devices are employed, because these instruments are relatively wide and straight and often difficult to align correctly with the uterine artery while also ensuring that the ureter is well clear of the tip of the instrument. It is therefore recommended either that the uterine artery is secured vaginally in these procedures, or that the ureter is identified and dissected away from the surgical field and the artery is then occluded with a suture or bipolar diathermy. If difficulty is encountered with identifying the ureter, a ureteric stent should be inserted before the operation proceeds any further.

Likewise, during oophorectomy in a previously hysterectomized patient, the ureter needs to be identified as it courses below the infundibulopelvic ligament and dissected free from the peritoneum on the pelvic sidewall to which the residual ovary is invariably adherent.

However, even using these techniques, the surgeon may be suspicious of ureteric damage during an operative procedure. If this is the case, 5 ml of indigo carmine solution can be injected intravenously. This will be excreted in the urine 5–10 min after injection and should highlight the site of ureteric damage. Any patient with postoperative loin pain should have an intravenous urogram performed; ultrasonography will fail to demonstrate dilatation of the renal pelvis in the immediate postoperative period.

Port closure and the prevention of hernia

As previously recommended, the secondary cannulae should be withdrawn under direct laparoscopic observation in case they have perforated a vessel in the anterior abdominal wall.

If a patient has a history of previous abdominal surgery, the surgeon should be alert to bowel adhering to the anterior abdominal wall and in particular under the site of the primary trocar.

Incisions in the peritoneum and those smaller than 10 mm in the rectus sheath will heal spontaneously, as will many skin incisions along Langer's lines. In larger incisions, used for large morcellating instruments, a deep absorbable suture should be inserted to close the deep fascia to prevent hernia formation. The use of the Phipps J-shaped needle (Rocket, London, UK) or EndoClose (Auto Suture, Ascot, UK) is necessary to ensure adequate closure of the fascial layer. Hernias appear to be more common at the site of the laterally placed incisions. Approximation of the skin can be achieved using Steri-strips (St Pauls, Minnesota, USA) and/or absorbable or non-absorbable sutures.

Adhesiolysis

The causes of adhesions continue to be poorly understood, although the problems resulting from them are better defined except in their relationship with pain.

Adhesions are potentially challenging to the operative laparoscopist. They tempt most surgeons to intervene surgically, and this can be a hazardous route to take. Adhesiolysis of fine postinfective adhesions around the tube and ovary may be one of the easiest laparoscopic operations. Adhesiolysis of dense endometriotic and bowel adhesions, on the other hand, will challenge the surgeon's ability and these are among the most difficult procedures to perform, with a high rate of complication. As always, the surgeon should resist the temptation to cut or free adhesions unless there is a definite correlation between the adhesions and the patient's symptoms.

There are three basic indications for adhesiolysis: to facilitate access to the organs the surgeon intends to operate on, to dissect adhesions causing infertility, and to free adhesions in patients complaining of altered bowel function. One must remember that adhesions tend to recur, although there is evidence that this is less of a problem with a laparoscopic approach.

Various methods have been proposed to reduce the formation of adhesions following laparoscopic surgery. The methods we employ are to achieve meticulous haemostasis and to wash blood and debris from the peritoneal cavity at the end of the procedure. We leave approximately 300 ml of Ringer's lactate in the pelvis, and if any large areas of peritoneum have been dissected Interceed (Johnson and Johnson, Slough, UK) is placed over these areas.

Summary

Laparoscopic management of ectopic pregnancy, simple ovarian cysts, mild or moderate endometriosis and pelvic infection should now be the norm, and will soon be demanded by patients.

In experienced hands, the complication rate of operative laparoscopy should be no greater than that for diagnostic laparoscopy or conventional surgery. Specialized training gives an increased awareness of how to avoid complications and to diagnose complications as they occur. It is therefore as relevant to the occasional diagnostic level 1 laparoscopist as to the level 4 advanced laparoscopic surgeon.

The majority of complications associated with laparoscopic surgery occur as a result of the creation of a pneumoperitoneum and the blind insertion of the primary trocar. These complications are complications of the laparoscopic *approach* and not the laparoscopic *technique*.

Acknowledgements

Parts of this text are taken from McMillan and Harding (1994) and McMillan *et al.* (1994). They are reproduced here with the permission of their respective publishers, Churchill Livingstone and Radcliffe Medical Press.

Bibliography

Baadsgaard SE, Bill S, Egeblad K. (1989) Major vessel injury during gynaecological laparoscopy. Report of a case and review of published cases. *Acta Obstet Gynecol Scand* **68**: 283–5.

Baggish MS, Lee WK, Miro SJ, Dacko L, Cohen G (1979) Complications of laparoscopic sterilization. *Obstet Gynecol* **54**: 54–9.

Chamberlain G, Brown JD (eds) (1978) *Gynaecologic Laparoscopy. Report of the Confidential Enquiry into Gynaecologic Laparoscopy.* Royal College of Obstetricians and Gynaecologists, London.

Copeland C, Wine RR, Hulka JF (1983) Direct trocar insertion at laparoscopy. *Obstet Gynecol* **62**: 655–9.

DeCherney AH (1985) The leader of the band is tired. *Fertil Steril* **44**: 299.

Hasson HM (1974) Open laparoscopy: a report of 150 cases. *J Reprod Med* **12**: 234–8.

Holtz G (1987) Laparoscopy in the massively obese female. *Obstet Gynecol* **69**: 423–4.

Howard FM (1992) Breaking new ground or just digging a hole? An evaluation of gynaecologic operative laparoscopy. *J Gynaecol Surg* **8**: 143.

Krebs HB (1986) Intestinal injury in gynecologic surgery: a ten year experience. *Am J Obstet Gynecol* **155**: 509–14.

McMillan DL, Harding SG (1994) Gynaecological endoscopic surgery. In: Clements RV (ed.) *Safe Practice in Obstetrics and Gynaecology*. Churchill Livingstone, London, pp. 321–35.

McMillan DL, Harding SG, Pesce A (1994) Complications of gynaecological endoscopy. In: Grochmal S (ed.) *Minimal Access Gynaecology*. Radcliffe Medical Press, Oxford.

Nezhat C, Nezhat F, Nezhat C (1992) Operative laparoscopy (minimally invasive surgery). State of the art. *J Gynecol Surg* **8**: 111.

Peterson HB, Halfa JF, Philip JM (1990) American Association of Gynaecologic Laparoscopists. 1988 membership survey on operative laparoscopy. *J Reprod Med* **35**: 587–9.

RCOG (1994) *Report of the RCOG Working Party on training in gynaecological endoscopic surgery*. Royal College of Obstetricians and Gynaecologists, London.

Yuzpe AA (1990) Pneumoperitoneum needle and trocar injuries in laparoscopy. *J Reprod Med* **35**: 485–90.

Chapter 8

Principal Laparoscopic Operative Techniques

S.P. Ewen

Introduction

Minimal access gynaecological surgery has undergone rapid development in the last 5 years, during which time there has been a similarly dramatic increase in the range of instrumentation available for use at operative laparoscopy. This chapter reviews the principal laparoscopic techniques for cutting, suturing and achieving haemostasis, including an overview of the instrumentation available.

Cutting

Scissors

Reusable laparoscopic scissors usually have one fixed blade and one moving blade. They are available in a variety of styles, hook scissors being the most commonly used (Figure 8.1). A major problem and source of frustration is that these reusable scissors invariably become blunt quickly. Disposable scissors overcome this problem and their extra costs are well worth while. They can also be connected to monopolar diathermy equipment to achieve haemostasis while cutting.

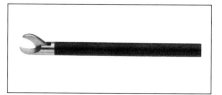

Figure 8.1 *Hook scissors (courtesy of Karl Storz, Tuttlingen, Germany).*

Diathermy applicator

Continuous unipolar cutting current applied through a 1 mm diathermy needle electrode (Figure 8.2) can provide fairly precise cutting, although there will be lateral thermal tissue damage[1] of up to 1 mm, which is not as precise as the carbon dioxide laser. (Lasers are considered later in this chapter.) The sharp edge of a hook or spatulated electrode will also provide effective cutting.

Harmonic scalpel

This device consists of a disposable blade that vibrates at 55 000 times a second, which in contact with tissue causes cutting and coagulation. It provides little advantage over scissors.

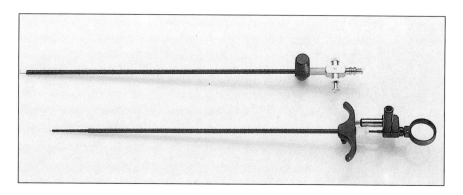

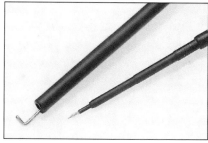

Figure 8.2 *Hook and needle electrode for unipolar diathermy.*

Haemostasis

There are a variety of techniques that can be chosen to secure vessels and vascular pedicles, depending on the clinical situation, availability, cost and individual preference (Table 8.1).

Unipolar diathermy

Unipolar cutting current can achieve coagulation of small and moderate-sized vessels by using a larger electrode surface, thereby lowering the power density. The most practical application of this phenomenon is to use the larger flat side of the scissors held in contact with the tissue to coagulate before cutting. Pure cutting current can be modified using a blend setting, thereby interrupting the continuous current. The interrupted waveform is of a higher voltage than the cutting waveform and provides more tissue destruction and resultant haemostasis.

Bipolar diathermy

The electrical current passes from one electrode to another and returns to the electrosurgical generator. Tissue present between the electrodes (the blades of the bipolar forceps, Figure 8.3) is heated and undergoes coagulation. Large vessels, such as the ovarian and uterine vessels, can be secured with this method. A practical problem is determining the optimum time for application of the current. If this is too short, bleeding will occur when the vessel is cut; if tissue is coagulated excessively, the bipolar forceps will stick to the tissue and tear it when removed. These problems can be overcome by incorporation of an ammeter in the system, which detects when current ceases to flow between the bipolar forceps blades, indicating that coagulation is complete and the pedicle can be safely cut. The electrosurgical generator Erbotom ACC 455 (ERBE Electromedizin, Tübingen, Germany) has this autobipolar facility and is of particular value in advanced laparoscopic surgery.

Table 8.1 *Advantages and disadvantages of techniques for haemostasis*

Technique	Advantages	Disadvantages
Staples	Quick and easy	Cost
	Reliable	12 mm instrument
Sutures	Cheap	Time consuming
		Technically difficult
Bipolar diathermy	Cheap	Slower than staples
	5 mm instrument	Lateral thermal spread
Unipolar diathermy	Versatile	Small vessels only
		Unipolar risks

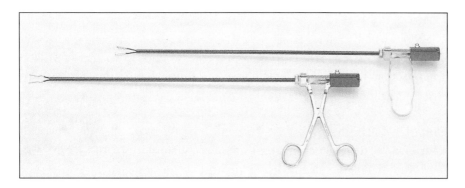

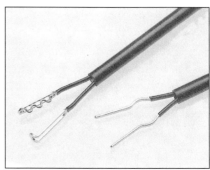

Figure 8.3 *Bipolar forceps.*

Argon beam coagulator

The argon beam coagulator (Figure 8.4) provides a unipolar spray coagulation current activated within a stream of argon gas. The advantage over conventional unipolar diathermy is that the argon gas ionizes and facilitates current flow between the instrument and tissue, allowing a bigger distance between the electrode and the tissue. Furthermore, the gas blows blood and debris away from the target area allowing direct fulguration of the bleeding vessels. High flow rates of argon gas are potentially dangerous, carrying a risk of embolism and abdominal gas evacuation is vitally important. The argon beam coagulator is particularly useful for achieving haemostasis of vascular beds such as after myomectomy.

Clips and staples

Individual clips may be useful to achieve haemostasis; however, the vessels must be skeletonized to enable application of the clips, which may be absorbable (e.g. PDS, Absolock clips, Ethicon, Edinburgh, UK) or inert titanium clips within an automatic clip applicator (e.g. EndoClip, Auto Suture, Ascot, UK; Ligaclip, Ethicon).

Haemostatic stapling devices (Figure 8.5) are very effective for securing and ligating vascular pedicles during operative laparoscopy, and are particularly useful during laparoscopic hysterectomy. Models are available from both Auto Suture (EndoGIA) and Ethicon (Endopath Linear Cutter, ELC). They are inserted down a 12 mm cannula and have a cartridge consisting of three rows of titanium staples either side of a knife blade. The staple rows are arranged as illustrated in Figure 8.6 to provide haemostasis, and the blade divides the tissue between them. Two cartridge types are available: blue for thicker tissue and white for thin vascular pedicles. In my experience, it is rarely necessary to use blue cartridges, and haemostasis is very much more reliable with the white vascular cartridge.

Once the tissue has been closed into a jaw of the stapler it is essential to ensure that no unwanted structures are included, such as ureter, bladder or bowel. The gun is fired, the staples are thus inserted,

Figure 8.4 *(a) Argon beam coagulator. (b) The argon gas provides an electron channel allowing monopolar current to impinge directly on a bleeding vessel.*

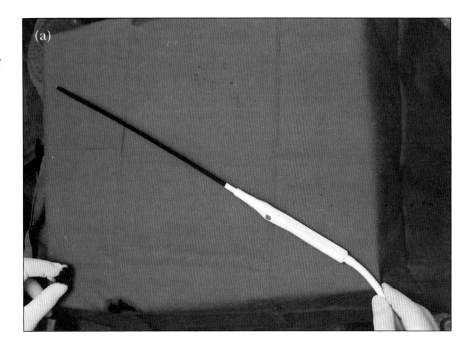

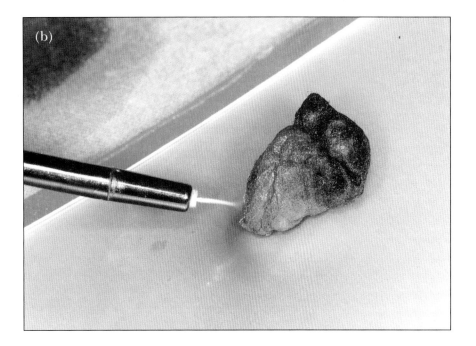

and the knife blade cuts the tissue between the two rows of staples (Figure 8.7). These devices are quick and effective; however, initially, there were reports of damage to the ureter[2] during laparoscopically assisted vaginal hysterectomy. Great care must be taken when securing the uterine vessels using these stapling devices to ensure that the ureter is not damaged.

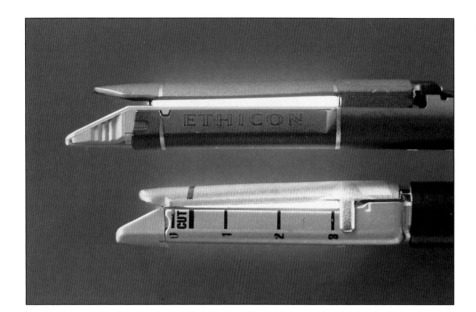

Figure 8.5 *Stapling devices.*

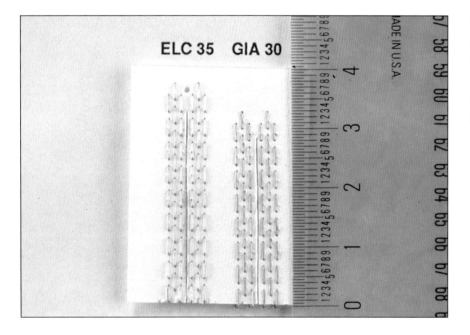

Figure 8.6 *Three rows of titanium staples are inserted either side of a knife blade, which automatically cuts the tissue in between. The Ethicon device is 5 mm longer than the EndoGIA.*

Sutures

Although suturing at laparoscopy can be frustrating and time consuming, surgeons undertaking operative laparoscopy should be skilled in suturing as this may be essential in certain circumstances to achieve haemostasis. Laparoscopic suturing may be performed within the abdomen (intracorporeal) or the surgical knots may be formed outside the abdomen and pushed down into place (extracorporeal).

Figure 8.7 *Use of staples during laparoscopically assisted vaginal hysterectomy.*

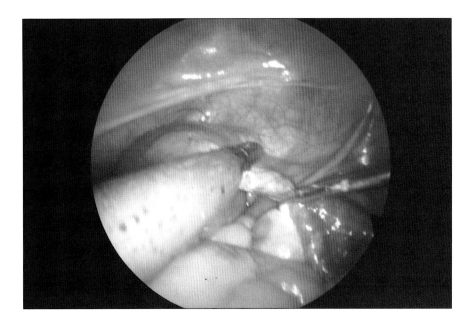

Extracorporeal suturing

The Endoloop technique (Figure 8.8) was first described by Semm[3] and involves securing pedicles with pre-tied Roeder loops. The structure to be secured is brought through the centre of the loop, and the knot is then tightened and pushed down with the plastic pusher. This technique is relatively simple and can be useful in a number of situations, for example salpingectomy. For safety, three loops are generally used. Alternatively, individual throws can be pushed down with a knot pusher to secure a knot while maintaining tension from above. To prevent excessive loss of gas during this technique, a trocar without a trap valve is preferable, for example the Hunt–Reich trocar.

The Endoknot (Ethicon) and Surgi-whip (Auto Suture) devices consist of a suture running through a plastic knot pusher at one end of its length with a needle attached at the other end (Figure 8.9) to enable passing of a suture through the tissue before tying it. Many surgeons find either straight or ski-shaped needles easier to manipulate than curved needles, and these tend to be more commonly available. In addition to securing vascular pedicles, this type of suture may be useful to approximate tissue, for example in repairing a hole in the bladder.

If the suture is grasped close to the base of the needle, it can be passed down a 5 mm trocar into the abdomen. Using a needle holder, the needle is passed through the tissue and then removed through the same trocar. A Roeder slip knot (Figure 8.10) is tied and pushed down into position to secure the suture. Alternatively a suture of choice without incorporated knot pusher may be used in the same way, and

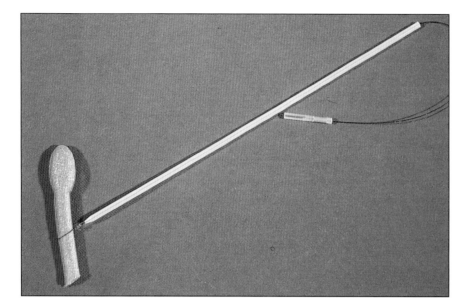

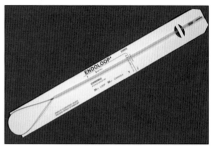

Figure 8.8 *Endoloop loop with pre-tied Roeder knot.*

Figure 8.9 *Endoknot.*

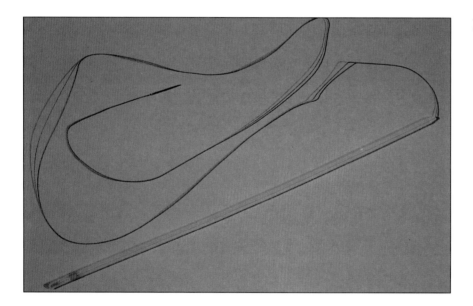

the Roeder knot pushed down with a dedicated instrument such as the Clarke–Reich knot pusher (Marlow Surgical, USA).

Intracorporeal suturing

This technique involves tying the knot within the abdomen. If a similar small straight or ski-shaped needle is used it can be introduced via a 5 mm cannula as previously described. If a larger curved needle is used, a 10 or 12 mm cannula may be necessary or, alternatively, the needle can be inserted using the technique described by Reich *et al.*[4], which enables needle insertion into the abdomen via a 5 mm incision.

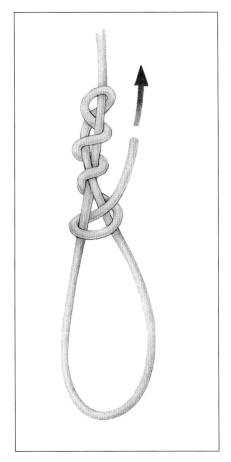

Figure 8.10 *Roeder knot. A single throw is made with the two suture ends, the knot being held with the thumb and third finger of the left hand. The free end is looped three times round both suture strands, the tail of the suture inserted through the last loop formed, and the knot pulled tight.*

The 5 mm cannula is removed from the abdomen, and an assistant places a finger over the incision to prevent gas leak. The distal end of the suture is back-loaded through the cannula, then the needle holder is reinserted through the cannula and the suture grasped near the base of the needle. The needle holder is then inserted through the existing 5 mm incision and down the path where the cannula was previously sited, thus pulling the needle through into the abdomen. The cannula is then reinserted over the needle holder.

It is important to select a short length of suture for intracorporeal knot tying to prevent excess length complicating the procedure. It is desirable to use two needle holders to manipulate the needle within the abdomen.

Endostitch

This ingenious device from Auto Suture (Figure 8.11) simplifies the loading and manipulation of needles and sutures. The needle has the suture attached in the middle and can pass from arm to arm of the needle holder through tissue. Intracorporeal knot tying is also considerably simplified. It is not suitable for use in sites where access is limited, as in colposuspension techniques; however, it is very useful for tissue approximation such as repairing peritoneal defects and cystotomy.

Lasers

Lasers are by no means essential for operative laparoscopy, but are an extremely useful and safe tool. The lasers most commonly used in gynaecology are the carbon dioxide, neodymium yttrium aluminium garnet (Nd-YAG) and potassium titanyl phosphate (KTP) lasers. The properties of these lasers are compared in Table 8.2.

Carbon dioxide

Professor Bruhat and his team at Clermont-Ferrand[5] were the first to report the use of carbon dioxide laser laparoscopy in gynaecology in 1979. This laser provides energy at a wavelength of 10 600 nm, an invisible light laser within the infrared area of the spectrum. The laser beam is delivered via a rigid arm containing a series of aligned mirrors. The laser results in high energy impact, producing intense heat and vaporization of cell contents. Because it is strongly absorbed by water, and the majority of biological tissue volume is water, penetration of this laser is limited[6] to 70 μm. As a result of these properties, the laser is a tool of tremendous precision, ideal for the vaporization of endometriosis overlying vital structures, or for performing salpingolysis. In ultrapulse mode, the laser can give precise char-free cutting with tissue damage limited[1] to 50 μm.

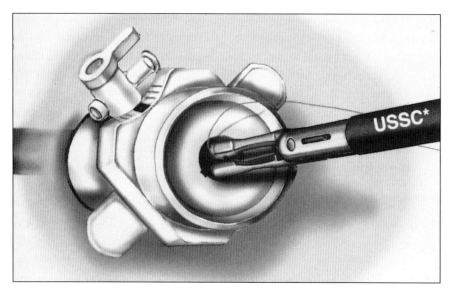

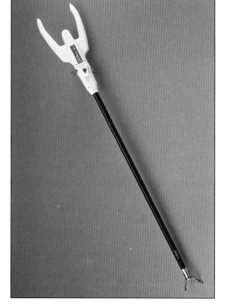

Figure 8.11 *EndoStitch (courtesy of Auto Suture, Ascot, UK).*

Table 8.2 *Properties of surgical lasers*

	Carbon dioxide	Nd-YAG	Diode	KTP
Wavelength (mm)	10 600	1064	810	532
Primary tissue effect	Vaporization	Coagulation	Coagulation	Coagulation
Scattering of beam	None	Extensive	Slight	Slight
Effect on water	Strongly absorbed	Slightly absorbed	Not absorbed	Not absorbed
Fibre transmission	No	Yes	Yes	Yes
Depth of tissue effect (mm)	0.1	4–5	2–3	1–2

Smoke is produced and needs to be evacuated from the abdomen to maintain clear vision. As the energy is absorbed by fluid, this laser becomes useless in the presence of fluid or blood and will not prevent bleeding other than from capillary vessels. The laser beam may be delivered via an operating laparoscope or via specially designed probes through a second port. The choice of technique employed depends largely on the preference of the operator.

Nd-YAG

This laser produces a wavelength of 1064 nm, and is delivered via optical fibres. Tissue penetration is significant (3–5 mm) and scatter is extensive, leading to excellent coagulation ideal for endometrial ablation. However, during laparoscopic surgery, the Nd-YAG laser is

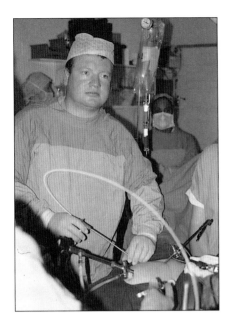

Figure 8.12 *The KTP laser produces an emerald green beam, which is passed down a flexible fibre.*

unsafe to use via a bare fibre because of extensive penetration and scatter, which may damage underlying structures. To overcome this problem, sapphire tips and sculptured quartz tip fibres have been produced, which concentrate the laser beam energy. This produces intense heating of the tip, and cutting or coagulation is purely a thermal effect rather than a laser tissue reaction such as vaporization. A major disadvantage of these special fibres and tips is that they are very expensive. When using the Nd-YAG laser, protective safety goggles have to be worn by all theatre personnel because the wavelength can permanently damage the macular part of the retina.

KTP

In this laser, energy is generated by an Nd-YAG laser and passed through a KTP crystal, thereby halving the wavelength and producing energy at 532 nm. It is an emerald green visible light laser (Figure 8.12) that penetrates tissue to a depth of 1–2 mm. It is safe to use at laparoscopy, although it is not as precise as the carbon dioxide laser, but has the advantage that the light can be passed down flexible fibres and will work in the presence of fluid. The wavelength is close to the absorption peak of haemoglobin and thus the laser tissue interaction is particularly suitable for photocoagulation in endometriosis and endometriomas. A major advantage of the KTP laser over the Nd-YAG laser is that specially designed tips are not necessary. Standard quartz fibres are used, to incise or vaporize tissue by touching, or to cut by dragging the fibre over the tissue. Coagulation can be achieved by moving the fibre further away from the tissue.

Argon

The Argon laser is a visible blue-green beam at 488 nm. It is similar to the KTP laser but is power limited and does not cut as effectively.

Diode

Diode lasers capable of producing power at surgically useful levels have recently been developed (Figure 8.13). Among the best is the Diomed laser. It uses laser energy at a wavelength of 810 nm via a flexible quartz fibre. The first release was limited to a power of 25 W. This has recently been upgraded to 60 W and is useful for endometrial ablation and large-scale tissue vaporization. It has similar properties to the Nd-YAG laser, but penetrates less deeply while still coagulating tissue effectively. Its main advantage is its portability, rugged solid-state construction and very low maintenance costs. These lasers may represent the next wave of laser technology.

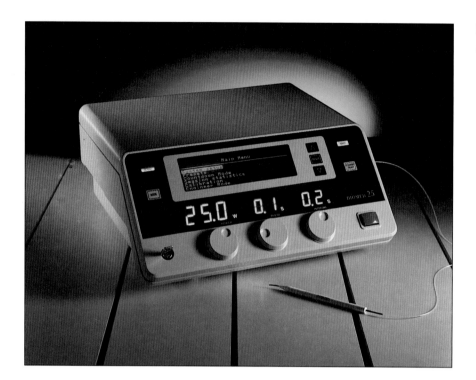

Figure 8.13 *The Diomed 25 surgical diode laser.*

Summary

There are many different techniques and instruments that can be used during operative laparoscopy to achieve the principal effects of cutting and haemostasis. Automated stapling or clip devices are quick, easy to use and reliable but unfortunately expensive; sutures are cheap but more time consuming. The majority of procedures can be achieved with unipolar and bipolar electrodiathermy, but for precision the carbon dioxide laser is superior.

The choice of tool is less important than the training and experience of the surgeon holding the tool, in the properly selected patient.

References

1. Sutton CJG, Hodgson R (1992) Endoscopic cutting with lasers. *Minimal Invasive Therapy* **1**: 197–205.
2. Woodland MB (1992) Ureter injury during laparoscopy: assisted vaginal hysterectomy with the endoscopic linear stapler. *Am J Obstet Gynecol* **167**: 756–7.
3. Semm K (1986) Operative pelviscopy. *Br Med Bull* **42**: 284–95.
4. Reich H, Clarke HC, Sekel L (1992) A simple method for ligating in operative laparoscopy with straight and curved needles. *Obstet Gynecol* **79**: 143–7.

5. Bruhat M, Mages C, Manhes H (1979) Use of CO_2 laser via laparoscopy. In: Kaplan I (ed.) *Laser Surgery III. Proceedings of the third congress of the International Society for Laser Surgery.* Jerusalem Press, Tel Aviv, pp. 275–81.

6. Baggish MS (1980) High power density CO_2 laser therapy for early cervical neoplasia. *Am J Obstet Gynecol* **136**: 117–25.

Chapter 9

Principal Hysteroscopic Operative Techniques

G.H. Trew

Introduction

Background

Equipment

Procedures

Retrieval of intrauterine contraceptive devices
Endometrial biopsy
Polypectomy
Division of synechiae
Division of uterine septum

Summary

Introduction

This chapter reviews the major surgical modalities available in hysteroscopic surgery and provides practical guidelines for their safe introduction.

Background

With the advent of hysteroscopic surgery, many 'traditional' and certainly more invasive gynaecological procedures on the uterine corpus are now performed not only more quickly and less invasively but also more successfully and cheaply by hysteroscopic means. Before any form of hysteroscopic procedure is performed, though, surgeons must not only be competent and at ease performing diagnostic hysteroscopy, but must also understand what they are seeing. Variations on the normal uterine cavity are manifold and not necessarily pathological. Only by performing many diagnostic hysteroscopies will the surgeon realize what is pathological and what is normal.

There are three main surgical modalities used in hysteroscopic surgery: 'cold' instrumentation, electrosurgery and lasers. Each has its advantages and disadvantages (Table 9.1). Cold instrumentation is cheap to purchase and has low running costs, but some procedures can take longer to perform which increases theatre costs. The laser is expensive to purchase and to run, but the operating time can be shorter. Electrosurgery lies somewhere between the two in being relatively cheap to purchase and run, but also reasonably quick to use. It also has the bonus, along with cold instrumentation, of providing tissue for histological analysis in certain procedures.

Equipment

As with laparoscopic procedures, good equipment is extremely important. A video system (Figures 9.1 and 9.2) is preferable for diagnostic hysteroscopies but not essential, whereas for any form of hysteroscopic operation a video system is essential. The system not only gives a better view but also allows the hysteroscopist to sit in a more

	Cold	Electrosurgery	Laser
Expense	Low	Moderate	High
Length of procedure	Long	Short	Short
Histological specimen	Yes	Yes	No

Table 9.1 *Advantages and disadvantages of surgical modalities*

Figure 9.1 *Endovision Hysterocam video system (courtesy of Karl Storz, Tuttlingen, Germany).*

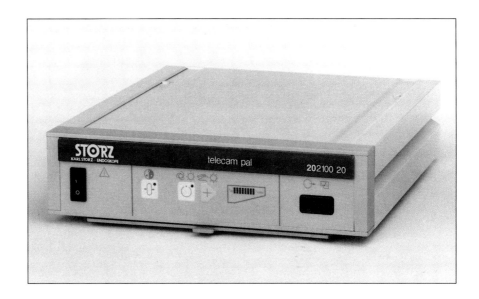

Figure 9.2 *Resectoscope with a Hysterocam camera system with free rotating head to keep a natural horizon on the monitor to facilitate orientation (courtesy of Karl Storz, Tuttlingen, Germany).*

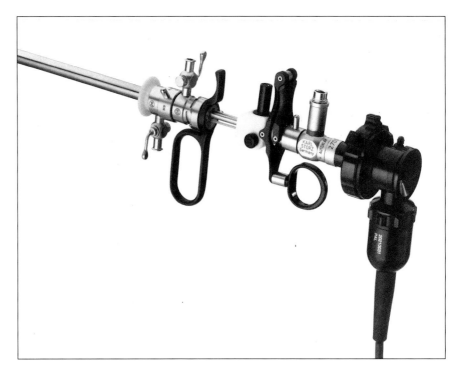

comfortable position for the longer procedures and hence take more time and care over them. A videohysteroscopic system also allows other colleagues in the operating theatre to view the proceedings and is mandatory if any teaching is taking place. Medicolegally, a video copy of the procedure is often helpful for the defence if a claim for negligence is pursued by the patient if there are later complications. Video recordings are also useful for teaching and comparing later findings with the original ones.

A modern light source (Figure 9.3) with a minimum power rating of 150 W is also mandatory. Performing any hysteroscopic procedure

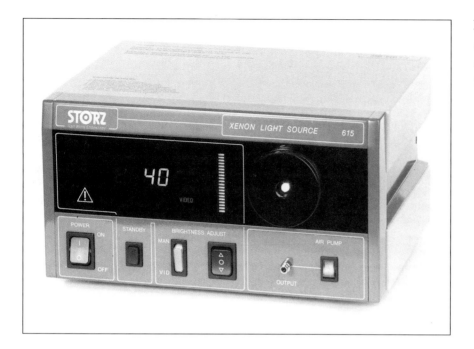

Figure 9.3 *Xenon light source suitable for laparoscopies and hysteroscopies (courtesy of Karl Storz, Tuttlingen, Germany).*

without adequate light and visualization is not only dangerous but frankly negligent.

Carbon dioxide, although an excellent medium for diagnostic hysteroscopy when used with a good insufflator (Figure 9.4), is not the medium of choice for any operative work. Some form of liquid medium is used: in the UK the majority of hysteroscopists use glycine. The medium has to be instilled into the cavity at a rate that allows adequate distension for visualization and clears any debris or blood, but not so high that problems such as the TURP (transurethral resection of the prostate) syndrome (see Chapter 10) arise. An

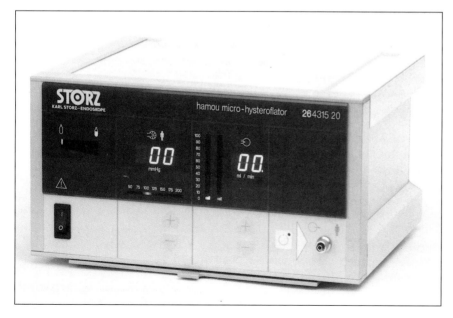

Figure 9.4 *Carbon dioxide insufflator for hysteroscopic use (courtesy of Karl Storz, Tuttlingen, Germany).*

Figure 9.5 *Irrigation pump for hysteroscopic or laparoscopic irrigation, set up for suction as well (courtesy of Karl Storz, Tuttlingen, Germany).*

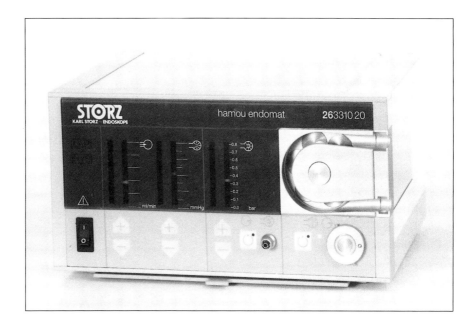

excellent pump for distension is shown in Figure 9.5; this has a dual function and can be used for both hysteroscopic distension and laparoscopic irrigation, thus cutting down on equipment costs.

A good quality hysteroscope should be available in all good theatre suites. Do not be tempted to use an old hysteroscope in the belief that all the other equipment will compensate for its inadequacies: hysteroscopes, like any other optical systems, deteriorate with repeated cleaning cycles and need to be replaced frequently depending on their usage.

A Hamou II continuous flow hysteroscope (Figure 9.6; Storz, Tuttlingen, Germany) has a diameter of 4 mm and can be used either in a 4.5 mm sheath (Figure 9.7) for diagnostic hysteroscopies (using carbon dioxide or fluid) or with a bridge (Figure 9.8) and operating sheath (external diameter 7 mm) for use with operating instruments. The sheath is inserted using the obturator as shown in Figure 9.9 or under direct vision. The operating channel of this bridge will accept a variety of semi-rigid instruments. Figure 9.10 shows a selection of the most useful tips. These instruments can perform the majority of procedures without extra equipment, and if the budget is limited these would be the optimal starting equipment.

Safety point

Hysteroscopy should never be performed using a carbon dioxide insufflator designed for laparoscopic use.

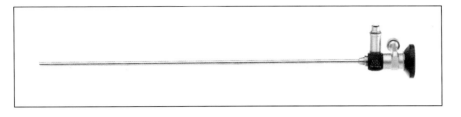

Figure 9.6 *Operating and contact hysteroscope. Forward-oblique 30° telescope, 4 mm external diameter.*

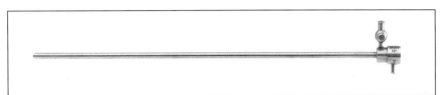

Figure 9.7 *45 mm examination sheath.*

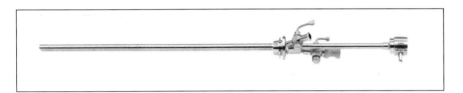

Figure 9.8 *Telescope bridge with operating channel for semi-rigid instruments.*

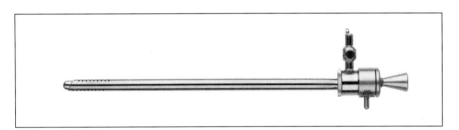

Figure 9.9 *7 mm operating sheath with obturator for assembly with the operating bridge illustrated in Figure 9.8.*

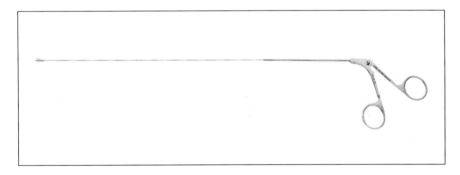

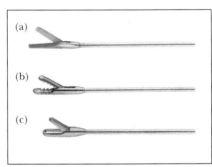

Figure 9.10 *Semi-rigid operating instruments, 7 Fr size: (a) scissors, (b) biopsy and grasping forceps, (c) biopsy forceps.*

The system required for hysteroscopic electrosurgery is quite different from that described above. Figures 9.2 and 9.11 show the assembled resectoscope, which can be used with a number of different electrodes. The various electrodes are shown in Figure 9.12 and the magnified tip of the scope with an angled cutting loop in Figure 9.13. The resectoscope should preferably be connected to one of the newer generation of diathermy machines (Figure 9.14) which have power settings for both cutting and coagulation. This allows more accurate and far safer cutting of tissue.

Figure 9.11 *Fully assembled resectoscope with electrode retracted.*

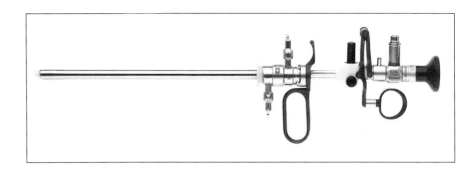

Figure 9.12 *Assorted electrodes: (a) cutting loop, angled, (b) coagulating electrode, 3 mm ball end, (c) coagulating electrode, 5 mm ball end, (d) coagulating electrode, 3 mm barrel end, (e) coagulating electrode, 5 mm barrel end, (f) coagulating electrode, pointed blade.*

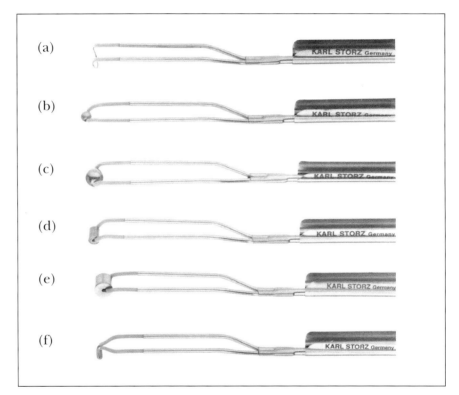

Figure 9.13 *Cutting electrode protruding from a resectoscope sheath.*

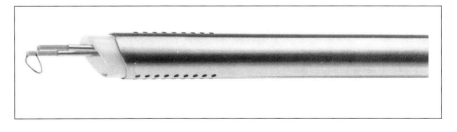

Figures 9.6–9.13 courtesy of Karl Storz, Tuttlingen, Germany

Laser energy can be used hysteroscopically as for electrosurgery. The most commonly used type is the Nd-YAG laser, but the newer diode lasers can also be used. (Carbon dioxide lasers are not suitable for hysteroscopic work.) The laser fibre is inserted through the operating channel of the hysteroscope (as in semi-rigid instruments) and manipulated by moving the fibre in the channel and/or the hysteroscope itself.

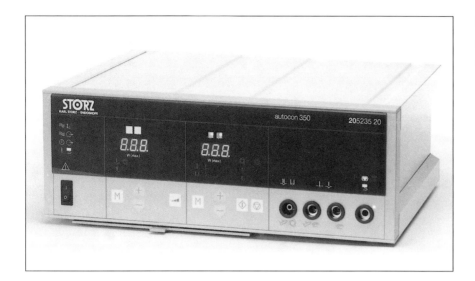

Figure 9.14 *High-frequency electrosurgical unit (courtesy of Karl Storz, Tuttlingen, Germany).*

Procedures

Many procedures can be performed hysteroscopically; some of the more commonly performed ones are listed below. Endometrial resection, laser endometrial ablation and hysteroscopic myomectomy will not be discussed in this chapter as they are covered very comprehensively in Chapters 15, 16 and 17, respectively.

Commonly performed hysteroscopic procedures

- Retrieval of intrauterine contraceptive devices
- Endometrial biopsy
- Polypectomy
- Division of synechiae
- Division of uterine septum
- Endometrial resection
- Laser endometrial ablation
- Hysteroscopic myomectomy

Retrieval of intrauterine contraceptive devices

The removal of an intrauterine contraceptive device (IUCD) when the strings have become detached or wrapped around it *in utero* is straightforward using a Hamou II hysteroscope and an operating bridge under direct vision. The device is held using the grasping forceps and the hysteroscope and the device removed as one unit from the cavity. Alternatively, if the strings are accessible in the cavity, these are grasped and drawn out of the cavity into the vagina, and the device is removed as normal. This procedure can be carried out as an outpatient procedure if a 2.5 mm flexible hysteroscope is used.

Endometrial biopsy

Blind curettage is notorious for missing abnormal uterine lesions. Hysteroscopic assessment of the cavity is not only a more thorough investigation but also allows any abnormal area to be visualized and a biopsy taken under direct guidance to ensure that the abnormal area is sampled and not a normal portion of the endometrium. The pick-up rates for hysteroscopically directed biopsy are far superior to those of blind sampling, either by dilatation and curettage or by outpatient sampling using one of the many cytological devices. The procedure is easily and rapidly performed either using the biopsy forceps and operating bridge or by taking a larger biopsy with the loop attachment to the resectoscope.

Polypectomy

Endometrial polyps are easily diagnosed hysteroscopically and can be easily removed for histological examination at the same session. They can be removed using the grasping forceps and the 7 mm scope or, if they are particularly large, using the resectoscope and cutting loop or blade. After the blade or loop has severed the base, the polyps can be extracted from the cavity using polyp forceps. If the base is large and bleeding is a problem, haemostasis can be achieved using a rollerball attachment as necessary.

Division of synechiae

Uterine synechiae are diagnosed either by hysteroscopy or by hysterosalpingography. Before operating, it is useful to give the patient some form of LHRH analogue to down-regulate the pituitary–ovarian axis and hence to put the patient into a temporary menopause and render her amenorrhoeic. This results in a very thin atrophic endometrium, which allows a far better view at hysteroscopy. It also reduces the amount of bleeding during the operation, which facilitates the procedure. We use goserelin (Zoladex, ICI Pharmaceuticals, Macclesfield, UK) and leuprorelin (Prostap-SR, Lederle, Gosport, UK; Figure 9.15) implants for either 1 or 2 months; both are very easy to give, and patient compliance is ensured. Danazol can also be used but has more side-effects, and so compliance may be a problem. The hysteroscope is introduced in the usual manner and the adhesions are divided as they are encountered in the cavity, preferably using semi-rigid scissors. (The diathermy blade or laser fibre can also be used.) Concurrent laparoscopy is not normally required although, if there is any doubt about what to cut and how much, laparoscopy can help. This happens particularly with dense cornual adhesions. After as many of the adhesions as possible have been divided, an IUCD is inserted.

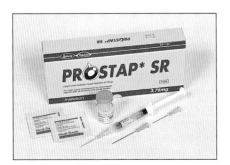

Figure 9.15 *Prostap-SR.*

After operation, a set regimen is always followed. This involves the administration of antibiotics, oestrogen and then progestogen as shown in Table 9.2. The IUCD is removed 6 weeks later and a hysterosalpingogram performed in the follicular phase of the next menstrual cycle after cessation of the next period. The patient is then reviewed as an outpatient to ascertain whether a further procedure is necessary.

Division of uterine septum

As with synechiae, uterine septa are diagnosed either by hysteroscopy or by hysterosalpingography. The preoperative work-up for septa is generally more extensive because of the varied anatomy possible and its congenital nature. Even if the septum is diagnosed at hysteroscopy, hysterosalpingography must always be performed. This gives a far better overall picture of the cavity and the defect itself; it is often difficult to assess the thickness of the septum from hysteroscopy alone. Laparoscopy must also be performed to differentiate between a partial bicornuate uterus and one with a partial septum, as this is impossible by hysterosalpingography or hysteroscopy alone (Figure 9.16). The same applies to diagnosis of complete septum and complete bicornuate uterus: only laparoscopically can the two be differentiated with any degree of certainty. Accurate diagnosis is necessary because of the subsequent treatment. Septum can be resected with excellent results, both anatomically and in terms of live birth rates. Partial bicornuate defects can sometimes be corrected, depending on the degree of the defect and the thickness of the fundal myometrium, but the surgeon must be very careful when resecting the defect to ensure that the full thickness of the wall is not cut. It is often helpful to perform the resection with simultaneous laparoscopy to visualize the cutting instrument as it approaches the visceral peritoneal surface of the uterus. Clear visualization also ensures that bowel is not lying over the uterine fundus where it may be damaged by heat transmitted during electrosurgery or laser surgery.

The septum is cut in a logical manner, caudally to cephalad, using any cutting method. Laser and electrosurgery tend to be quicker than

Table 9.2 *Standard drug regimes after division of synechiae*

	Week 1	Week 2	Week 3	Week 4
Antibiotics (cephalosporin and metronidazole)	1	2		
Oestrogen (Premarin (Ayerst, Maidenhead, UK) 0.625 mg daily)	1	2	3	
Progestogen (norethisterone 10 mg daily)			3	4

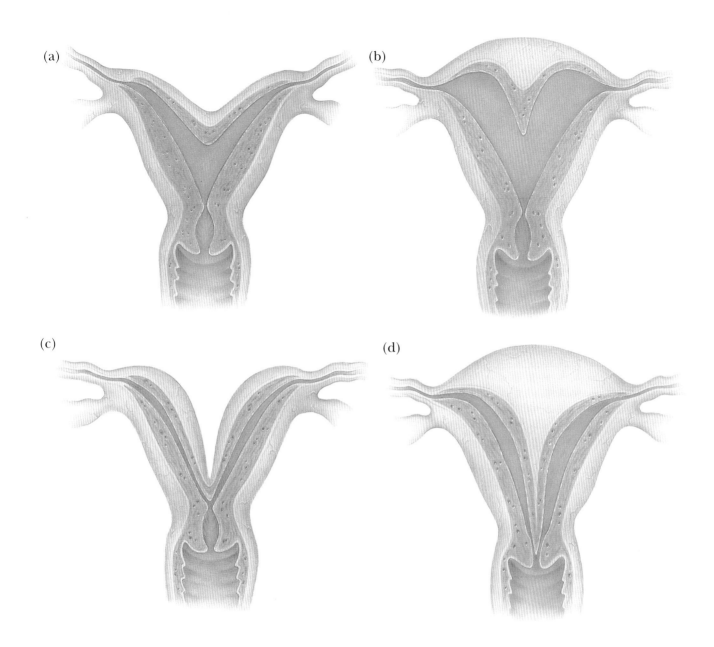

Figure 9.16 *Diagrammatic representation of (a) partial bicornuate uterus, (b) partial septate uterus, (c) complete bicornuate uterus, (d) complete septate uterus.*

scissors, particularly if the defect is large. Scissors are very exact but, because of the small bites of the blades, tend to take longer. Preoperative preparation with LHRH analogues is very helpful for resection, and the view obtained is markedly superior. The same postoperative regimen is followed as for synechiae, with the insertion of IUCDs and drug administration. If the septum has not been fully resected in the first session and two cavities are still present, however small the divide, two IUCDs are inserted – one in each cavity. It is not unusual with large septa to require a second operation to finish the division and separate any adhesions that may have formed. Attempting to complete the procedure in one operation increases the risk of fundal perforations with their sequelae.

Key points: division of uterine septum

- Hysterosalpingography must be performed
- Control laparoscopy is essential
- Endometrial suppression with an LHRH analogue is helpful
- Second-look hysteroscopy is advisable
- A two-stage procedure may be required

The patient should be warned to expect some bleeding and subsequent discharge but to return if the bleeding is heavy or the discharge offensive. If laser or electrosurgery has been used, the patient should also be warned to return if she experiences any vomiting, diarrhoea or abdominal pain. Bowel damage is unlikely if the procedure has been correctly performed, but the serious consequences and medicolegal aspects of bowel trauma make it sensible to be cautious and to warn the patient.

Summary

Improvements in fibre–optic systems and the ability to safely distend the uterine cavity have permitted the development of transcervical hysteroscopic operative techniques to treat conditions previously only accessible by open surgery. It is now possible under direct vision to remove an IUCD, perform an endometrial biopsy or polypectomy or excise synechiae and septa within the uterus. These procedures, once the appropriate skills have been acquired lead to more effective, safer treatment associated with a short duration of hospital stay and convalescence as well as an earlier return to normal activity.

Chapter 10

Hysteroscopic Complications and How to Avoid Them

O. Istre

Introduction

Complications of hysteroscopic surgery are often avoidable. This chapter outlines aspects of preoperative assessment of the patient that may reduce the risk of complications. The practical management of some of the more commonly encountered complications is addressed in detail.

Patient selection

Indications

Transcervical resection of the endometrium (TCRE) and of fibroids is an alternative to hysterectomy in dysfunctional bleeding. The operation is more likely to be successful if patients are carefully selected. Patients must be aware that childbearing cannot be considered[1] after TCRE. Treatment is more likely to be successful if the following criteria are satisfied.

Patient selection criteria

- Family complete
- Uterus smaller than 12 weeks gestational size
- Fibroids (submucous and <5 cm in diameter)
- Adenomyosis (limited or absent)
- Endometriosis (limited or absent)

The indications for TCRE are gradually evolving; in 1987 the indications for TCRE were considered by DeCherney to be contraindication to general anaesthesia, refusal to undergo hysterectomy and haemorrhagic disorders[2]. In 1991 there was general agreement favouring TCRE for menstrual symptoms justifying hysterectomy, which usually meant that conservative therapy had proved unsuccessful[1,3–5]. The uterus had to be of less than 12 weeks gestational size, and fibroids had to be submucous and smaller than 5 cm in diameter as indicated by ultrasonography or hysteroscopy. Women with other gynaecological diseases, like endometriosis and prolapse, were advised to have alternative treatment because of the probability of the need for further surgery[4]. Today, when more women are aware of the possibilities that new technology has created, there does not appear to be an absolute indication justifying hysterectomy. Many women suffer anaemia and menorrhagia for some time before accepting hysterectomy as the treatment of choice. These considerations will lead to further extension of the indications for TCRE.

Pathology

Uterine malignancy should be ruled out by means of preoperative cervical cytology and histological samples from the uterine cavity obtained by either the Pipelle Endocyt (Plurimed, Neuilly-en-Thelle, France) or the Vabra (Mediwise, Berkeley, California, USA) method[6]. These techniques usually provide a correct diagnosis and an adequate specimen for histological analysis[7,8].

Removal of the endometrium has gained popularity in Europe because it allows double checking of endometrial histology. Malignancies of the endometrium have been detected in the specimens obtained from TCRE. In earlier studies, although women with irregular bleeding and postmenopausal bleeding were investigated prior to TCRE, four patients were found to have an unsuspected carcinoma of the endometrium after TCRE[9,10]. Most endometrial cancers have been diagnosed in postmenopausal women because this disease reaches a peak incidence in women aged between 65 and 74 years of age[11].

Women with atypical or adenomatous hyperplasia should not undergo TCRE because of the risk of later malignancy, as the preinvasive nature of endometrial hyperplasia is well established: the risk of malignancies with atypical hyperplasia[12] is 23% over 11 years. However, cystic glandular hyperplasia without atypia is not a contraindication for operation[13]. Women with cervical dysplasia can be treated in the usual fashion, and this condition is not a contraindication for TCRE.

Fibroids

Fibroids are the most frequent cause of menorrhagia. Their incidence in women with menorrhagia seems to be 20% when assessed by bimanual palpation[14]. A more accurate method of identifying fibroids is transvaginal ultrasonography[15] in conjunction with fluid instillation enhancing the specificity related to mapping of fibroids[16] (Figure 10.1). Hysteroscopy is able to detect uterine abnormality in a substantial number of patients with menorrhagia[17,18]. In our series of 412 patients undergoing TCRE after referral by general practitioners because of bleeding disturbance, fibroids were detected in 120 women (29%). Several aspects of fibroids in relation to TCRE have been debated, including the size of the uterus and fibroids. There is general agreement[4] that the uterus should be smaller than 12 weeks gestational size, the cavity less than 12 cm in length and the maximum size of intracavitary fibroids not more than 5 cm. These limitations seem to result from features of the equipment, both the resectoscope and the electrical sling being able to treat women safely and effectively

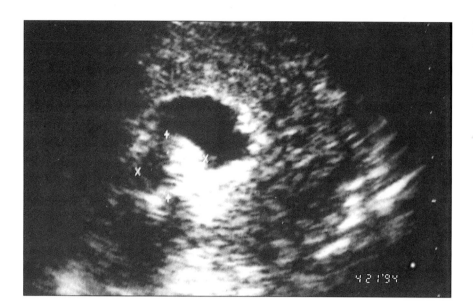

Figure 10.1 *Fluid-enhanced ultrasonogram showing a fibroid.*

only within these boundaries. Larger uteri or multiple fibroids should be effectively treated by another surgical approach, such as hysterectomy[19]. The location of the fibroid is another aspect to consider, complete resection improving the long-term results[20]. In marked intramural extension, different resection techniques should be applied. Thus, it is important to determine as much as possible about the fibroids before proceeding to surgery.

Ultrasonography

Transvaginal ultrasonography (TVS), as a non-invasive, accurate and cost-effective procedure, has become an indispensable investigation in modern gynaecological practice[21]. Selection of suitable preoperative cases with TVS may improve the success rate after transcervical resection of fibroids and thereby avoid additional surgery. In preoperative TVS performed on our patients, two parameters are assessed; the antero-posterior (AP) diameter and endometrial thickness (ET). The AP diameter is measured as it gives an excellent measurement of the size of the uterus. Smaller transverse and AP diameters of the uterus appear to predict a more successful outcome. Significant reduction in the AP diameter was measured in the successful group when assessed 3 months after operation[20] due to fibrosis and shrinkage. Peroperative problems with deficit of irrigation solution were more pronounced in patients with AP diameter >55 mm. The maximum double layer thickness of the endometrium (ET) was measured on a midline sagittal uterine section at the level of the maximum AP dimension of the uterus. An ET of <8.29 mm was significantly more often associated with amenorrhoea 1 year after TCRE.

A classification system for submucous fibroids on TVS has been developed. Pedunculated submucous fibroids without intramural extension are classified as type 0 fibroids. In type I, the submucous fibroid is sessile and the intramural part is less than 50%; with an intramural extension of 50% or more, the fibroid is classified as type II. The degree of intramural extension can be assessed by observing the angle of the fibroid with the endometrium at the attachment to the uterine wall[20]. Types I and II should be operated on with another technique and often require a repeat procedure.

Pelvic pain

A large number of patients suffer from pelvic pain. Three indications account for over half of the hysterectomies performed for non-malignant indications in the USA: leiomyomas, dysfunctional uterine bleeding and prolapse. A variable degree of pain is an indication for surgery in these women[22]. Pelvic pain that originates outside the uterus, caused by endometriosis and adhesions, will not be relieved by TCRE and may require another approach in both diagnosis and treatment. Although diagnosis and explanation for the pain may be difficult, TCRE or removal of fibroids has been beneficial whether or not menorrhagia has accompanied the dysmenorrhoea[4]. In our own series menstrual pain was reduced after TCRE.

Age

TCRE is irreversible and should be offered only to patients who have completed their families. This usually means that only patients older than 25 years should be offered TCRE for fibroids. (The age of 25 years is the age for legal sterilization in Scandinavian countries.) The prevalence of menorrhagia is lowest in young women and highest at 45 years. High parity is also associated with an increased incidence of menstrual disorders[23].

TCRE can be considered in some cases of post menopausal bleeding, however preoperative endometrial biopsies are mandatory. In our study of 412 patients undergoing TCRE, 13 of these patients were more than 55 years of age. The preoperative histology in this group was hyperplasia (six), polyps (four), secretory (one), proliferative (one) and atropic endometrium (one). This was confirmed in the specimen obtained at operation. These findings are in accordance with those of Brooks *et al.*, who performed TCRE in 26 patients aged 50 years and older[24]. These findings and my own experience indicate that an upper age limit for TCRE is not necessary.

Operative complications

Perforation

The most dangerous complication during hysteroscopic surgery is perforation, possibly damaging adjacent organs. In larger series of

---

Operative complications

- Perforation
- Absorption of distension medium
- Haemorrhage
- Infection

TCRE the incidence of perforation is small. Magos reported four perforations in 250 patients and Rankin two in 400 patients[4,10]. In our series of 412 patients nine perforations occurred, significantly more perforations occurring in the first 50 patients[3] than in the rest of the series. In perforation during hysteroscopy, laparotomy seems to be unnecessary; our patients have been observed in the ward for complications, and apart from the perforation no complications were encountered in any of the women. Bowel injury is the most feared and difficult complication after TCRE. It is believed to be caused by direct damage by the resectoscope on the bowel surface[25,26], although in most of the reports bowel injury occurs during ablation techniques using rollerballs and Nd-YAG lasers[27,28]. During ablation there is an immediately visible thermal injury of 5 mm depth, and even more when the energy source is maintained at the same spot for too long[29-31]. An intrauterine pressure of about 100 mmHg was used during hysteroscopic surgery in our patients to achieve sufficient distension of the cavity. The intestines are probably flushed away in the event of perforation, with immediate cooling of the resection sling[3]. Finishing the operation after a perforation can be difficult, but in the absence of major intra-abdominal trauma the perforation may be sutured by laparoscopy and the resection can be continued[32].

Absorption of irrigation medium

Complications include transurethral resection of the prostate (TURP) syndrome, which is a clinical entity related to massive absorption of the irrigating solution[33,34]. Although toxic effects of glycine and its metabolites may contribute to the syndrome, absorption of water, with dilutional hyponatraemia (Figure 10.2), water intoxication, cerebral oedema and cardiac overload, is considered to be a main characteristic of the syndrome[35-38]. Absorption of the irrigating medium is presumably related to the intrauterine pressure applied during the procedure. In our patients, a maximum pressure of about 100 mmHg was applied to the infusion system, but the pressure fall along the infusion line and the application of suction to the effluent makes the intrauterine pressure difficult to assess. The actual pressure probably exceeds the low levels recommended during resection of the

Figure 10.2 *Serum sodium ion level immediately after operation in 412 patients.*

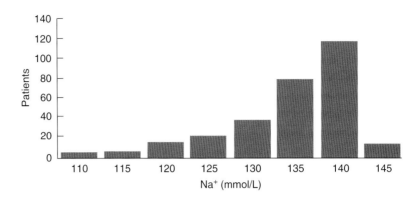

prostate[34], but the periprostatic venous sinuses have no equivalent within the myometrium.

The results of our study suggest that, provided there is sufficient peroperative control of the deficit, pressures up to 100 mmHg can be applied within the uterine cavity without occurrence of marked TURP syndrome-like complications. We have demonstrated marked changes of coagulation parameters after absorption of significant amounts of the glycine solution. Although the decrease seen in the levels of thrombocytes, haptoglobin and fibrinogen may be partly explained by simple dilution, absorption of the hypo-osmotic glycine solution (about 200 mOsmol/l) may cause some degree of haemolysis as well. Moreover, the increased levels of D-dimers probably reflect activated coagulation states associated with continuous and latent formation of thrombin and the onset of reactive fibrinolysis. Such changes are common after major operative procedures and seem to occur after TCRE as well[39]. These changes seem, however, to have little clinical implication.

During TCRE with 1.5% glycine as irrigation solution, about one in three patients experience postoperative nausea[40]. The patients suffering from such discomfort had all absorbed significant amounts of glycine, together with the water solvent, leading to plasma levels ranging from 5000 to 18 000 μmol/l (normal plasma levels 110–330 μmol/l). Glycine is the simplest of all amino acids and undergoes a variety of metabolic reactions, largely of a synthetic nature. The conversion to serine is one of the dominant pathways when there is an excess of glycine available[41]. Thus, the finding that the plasma serine level of patients with nausea is high several hours after surgery is probably due to the conversion of glycine to serine. The secondary excess of serine may interact with cystathionine leading to increased cysteine. The plasma concentration of ten other amino acids, including glycine, has been seen to increase. The high plasma levels of glycine and its secondary products may be responsible for some of the toxic symptoms observed after absorption of the irrigating glycine solution during TCRE. This absorption probably occurs mainly into vessels opened during the procedure, as no significant correlation between the peroperative glycine deficit and the operation time or the total amount of glycine used could be demonstrated in our study, in line with our earlier findings[40].

Patients with a glycine deficit of 1000 ml or more, or a decrease in serum sodium of 10 mmol/l or more, all experienced nausea and had a diagnosis of cerebral oedema on CT (Figure 10.3). The results suggest that discrete cerebral oedema may also contribute to the development of postoperative nausea in patients undergoing transcervical surgery with significant absorption of the glycine irrigating solution[42].

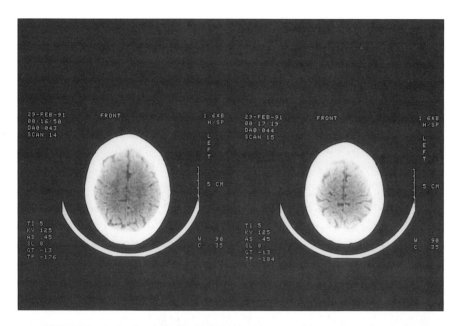

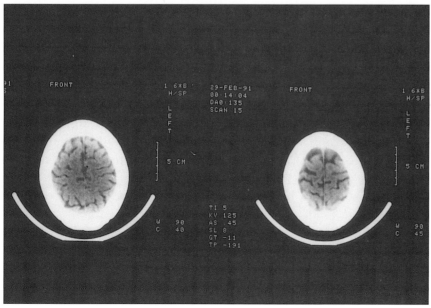

Figure 10.3 *Cerebral oedema on computed tomography.*

Although glycine 1.5% has been used traditionally for resectoscopic procedures, alternative irrigating solutions should now be actively sought. Moreover, the data available dictate cautious monitoring of the inflow pressure applied and the fluid absorption during transcervical resectoscopic surgery.

Features of TURP syndrome

● Dilutional hyponatraemia
● Thrombocytopenia
● Anaemia
● Hypofibrinogenaemia
● Cerebral oedema

Pathogenesis of TURP syndrome

● Absorption of water from irrigation medium
● Neurotoxicity caused by glycine and its metabolites
● Activated coagulation states

Haemorrhage

Peroperative heavy bleeding is uncommon during TCRE; Magos reported only one case in 250 patients who required uterine tamponade[4]. In the series of 400 consecutive patients of Rankin, peroperative excessive bleeding necessitating uterine tamponade was encountered in only four patients[10].

In a survey of the British Society for Gynaecological Endoscopy heavy bleeding during or after operation was reported in eight of 4038 patients[43]. In my own series of 412 TCRE operated patients peroperative heavy bleeding was encountered in 19 patients which necessitated tamponade by use of a Foley catheter chariere 24 filled with 30 ml of saline. The greater need for tamponade in these cases, compared with other series[4,10], could be due to the cautious approach of the author. On the other hand, it is a minor intervention and will certainly lead to the patient having a higher postoperative haemoglobin level.

Infection

Postoperative infection was defined as pain, malodorous discharge, fever >38 °C and increase in laboratory infection parameters. Infection was seen in 18 of 370 patients (4.9%) in our series. Five of these patients were readmitted to the hospital and treated with antibiotics, and the other 13 were treated on an outpatient basis. Peroperative prophylactic antibiotics were not given. In the survey from the British Society for Gynaecological Endoscopy 39 patients (1%) experienced different types of infection postoperatively, but the investigation did not remark on the use of prophylactic antibiotics[43]. As the questionnaire was sent only to the surgeons, some minor postoperative infections may have been treated by the local general practitioner without the gynaecologist's knowledge, thus leading to an underestimation of infections. The incidence of postoperative infection is modest and would not justify peroperative antibiotic prophylaxis in my opinion. However, patients who have a past history of pelvic inflammatory disease are at risk of developing infections, and prophylactic antibiotics during operative hysteroscopy appear to be effective in preventing infections in these patients[44].

Late complications of transcervical resection

Late complications

- Pain and persistent adenomyosis
- Haematometra
- Pregnancy
- Malignancy

Pain and persistent adenomyosis

Adenomyosis has been described as diagnostically elusive because of the difficulty of clinical identification and the unknown cause. It should be considered in all cases of menorrhagia and dysmenorrhoea, but remains asymptomatic in nearly half of all cases. Hysterectomy still remains the mainstay of diagnosis and treatment, although resectoscopic treatment has been proposed in some mild forms of adenomyosis to avoid hysterectomy. The adoption of standard histological criteria for adenomyosis seems important[45–47]. Adenomyosis is defined as the presence of endometrial glands in the myometrium without connection to the endometrial mucosa. The chips removed with the resectoscope seem to provide excellent specimens for histological examination. Thus, resection may offer an opportunity to make a reliable diagnosis of adenomyosis[48]. For this purpose, however, the resected specimens should be sliced perpendicular to the mucosal surface after fixation, preferentially in transverse sections, and oriented when embedded in paraffin. If treated in this way the carefully resected specimens will almost always constitute a useful tissue preparation for diagnostic purposes, obviously superior to the tissue fragments normally obtained by conventional curettage[49].

In our material, adenomyosis was found in the tissues resected from 94 (34.7%) of 271 patients who did not later have hysterectomy or re-resection. There were no differences between the group with or without adenomyosis in the menstrual bleeding pattern before or after the operation, 37 (39.4%) becoming amenorrhoeic in the group with adenomyosis. By contrast there were significant differences in the degree of preoperative pain in the these groups. 72 of 94 (77%) patients with histologically proven adenomyosis reported preoperative dysmenorrhea compared with 75 of 172 (44%) who did not have adenomyosis. Pain one year after TCRE was reduced to 11% and 13% respectively in these groups.

The incidence of adenomyosis is between 20 and 60%. Some authors have found that 40% of women undergoing TCRE have superficial adenomyosis[50]. More than 60% of patients with detectable adenomyosis suffer from meno/metrorrhagia and 30% complain of severe dysmenorrhoea – the classic symptom complex[51]. These observations agree with our observations, combinations of pain and menstrual bleeding problems being the main symptoms in patients with adenomyosis.

The reason for this improvement of preoperative pain following TCRE is hard to understand, but very often the reduction in bleeding intensity and pain goes together. It is possible that only minimal adenomyosis (adenomyosis sub-basalis (grade I), within one low-power field from the basalis) is adequately treated by TCRE[48]: the resectoscope removes 4 mm of the endometrium and myometrium and in this way all grade I adenomyosis is removed. Our data are in agreement with those of other authors, that minimal adenomyosis is not associated with adverse effects after TCRE[4]. By contrast, many cases of treatment failure, re-resection or subsequent hysterectomy showed evidence of more extensive invasion (grade II and III adenomyosis).

Haematometra and pain

Obstruction of the lower parts of the uterine cavity if the endometrium is active may lead to pain and haematometra[58]. The value of transvaginal ultrasonography in diagnosing postoperative pain caused by haematometra is obvious[21]. Appropriate treatment would be dilatation of the cervix or second-look resection with removal of residual endometrium. Fluid in the cavity after operation was seen in 15 of our patients; in only five of these was it accompanied by pain. It is difficult to decide using ultrasonography whether the fluid is haematometra coming from active endometrial tissue or not, but it is likely that patients with pain have small active endometrial glands. However, vaginal ultrasonography is useful in diagnosing cyclical postoperative pain and helpful in differentiating between haematometra and adenomyosis. Haematometra will benefit from dilatation; hysterectomy will be the treatment of choice in adenomyosis[21]. Follow-up after endometrial resection revealed a subgroup of women who developed late onset of pain with or without menstrual bleeding. We have observed that medroxyprogesterone acetate given at the time of surgery offers a continuing advantage in terms of patient satisfaction[59]. Of 164 patients operated on 24–60 months previously who received a questionnaire about satisfaction with the result of the operation, five (3%) reported *de novo* pain or worse pain than before operation. However, intolerable pain was the main indication for hysterectomy when TCRE had failed.

Tubal patency and pregnancy

Hysteroscopic sterilization by electrocoagulation is usually achieved during TCRE; previous investigations have shown a bilateral tubal occlusion rate of 80% confirmed by hysterosalpingography[52]. In the 1970s, there was great interest in methods to occlude the fallopian tubes at their uterotubal ostia, the potential advantages of a transcervical operation being avoidance of an abdominal incision and of possible adhesions. Electrocoagulation of the uterotubal ostia fell into disfavour because of failure to effectively occlude the ostia, apparently because of difficulties in locating the ostia and problems with the irrigation medium, current and equipment. We investigated tubal patency after TCRE hysterosalpingography and observed patent tubes in more than 10% of patients[53]. In a case report of a pregnancy after TCRE, the patient remained amenorrhoeic for 18 months after operation, but then an unexpected pregnancy occurred; in the operative description insufficient information about tubal coagulation with the rollerball was provided[54]. The risk of pregnancy after TCRE appears to be slight, although patients cannot be assured that this is a sterilization procedure. Other factors decreasing the possibility of nidation in the uterus include the reduced amount of endometrium, fibrosis and granulomatous inflammation. However, the potential for an abnormal outcome in a subsequent pregnancy is high[55,56]. Therefore, many authors recommend that a sterilization procedure be performed during the initial operation[1,57]. The need for another sterilization procedure may be overestimated particularly if operations can be scheduled postmenstrually and medication can be given before operation to reduce the thickness of the endometrium. Tubal occlusion can be confirmed by postoperative hysterosalpingography, although the incidence of recanalisation is uncertain.

Malignancy

Occlusion of the lower part of the cavity and the cervical canal may result in haematometra and pain, and may subsequently cause delay in the diagnosis of endometrial cancer. Cervical stenosis, fibrotic changes or synechiae may obstruct access to the cavity in some patients, and may delay the appearance of normal symptoms when malignancy of the remnants of the endometrium occurs. A major concern voiced by critics of TCRE is the possibility that endometrial adenocarcinoma may develop in crypts after ablation. One case of endometrial cancer following coagulation with the rollerball has been reported: the patient remained amenorrhoeic for 5 years before presenting with a 3 week history of moderate bleeding[60]. Vaginal ultrasonography may be of diagnostic value in such cases. A positive relation between endometrial thickness and endometrial cancer has been established, and no cases of endometrial abnormalities have been found when the endometrium was less than 5 mm thick[61]. However, the case mentioned above was a patient with a high risk for developing endometrial cancer and the procedure was a rollerball ablation. Until now no malignancies of the endometrium have been reported in patients who have undergone TCRE, but menstrual bleeding problems after TCRE should not be assumed to be treatment failures: endometrial carcinoma must be included in the differential diagnosis. Progestins should be added to hormone replacement regimens if HRT is indicated.

Summary

Surgical training is important when TCRE is performed: a significant number of operative complications can be anticipated in the first 20 procedures, reducing after 100 procedures.

TVS helps to identify uterine pathology and prognostic factors. Submucous fibroids make no difference to the clinical outcome of TCRE, but endometrial thickness does; there may be a useful role for agents that produce endometrial atrophy, or TCRE can be performed in the immediate postmenstrual phase of the cycle.

Nausea after TCRE is related to the deficit in glycine irrigant fluid, but not to the operation time or the total amount of irrigant fluid used, and may be partly explained by the toxic effects of glycine and its metabolites and by water intoxication and hyponatraemia. Plasma levels of glycine, nine other amino acids and ammonia are increased, and minor activation of fibrinolysis and haemolysis are also seen. Discrete cerebral oedema may also contribute to the development of postoperative nausea. We recommend that serum sodium levels be checked during the postoperative period, and indicate alternatives to glycine for irrigation solutions.

Tissue destruction and increase in uterine surface temperature are minimal during TCRE, and the procedure provides excellent histological material. Careful coagulation and resection in the cornual and isthmic regions are recommended. The uterine cavity after TCRE is narrow and fibrotic, but still accessible for diagnostic procedures. In most patients variable amounts of endometrium are found at second-look hysteroscopy and biopsy. Bleeding after TCRE may indicate endometrial carcinoma and should not be assumed to indicate treatment failure. Progestins should be added to the oestrogen replacement regimen. We recommend that tubal sterilization and TCRE be performed simultaneously; otherwise, these women must continue their normal contraceptive practice.

References

1 Ke RW, Taylor PJ (1991) Endometrial ablation to control excessive uterine bleeding. *Hum Reprod* **6**: 574–80.
2. DeCherney AH, Diamond MP, Lavy G, Polan ML (1987) Endometrial ablation for intractable uterine bleeding: hysteroscopic resection. *Obstet Gynecol* **70**: 668–70.
3. Istre O, Schiotz H, Sadik L, Vormdal J, Vangen O, Forman A (1991) Transcervical resection of endometrium and fibroids. Initial complications. *Acta Obstet Gynecol Scand* **70**: 363–6.
4. Magos AL, Baumann R, Lockwood GM, Turnbull AC (1991) Experience with the first 250 endometrial resections for menorrhagia. *Lancet* **337**: 1074–8. [erratum appears in *Lancet* **337** (1991) 1362; see comments]
5. McLucas B (1991) Intrauterine applications of the resectoscope. *Surg Gynecol Obstet* **172**: 425–31.
6. Chambers JT, Chambers SK (1992) Endometrial sampling: When? Where? Why? With what? *Clin Obstet Gynecol* **35**: 28–39.
7. Stovall TG, Ling FW, Morgan PL (1991) A prospective, randomized comparison of the Pipelle endometrial sampling device with the Novak curette. *Am J Obstet Gynecol* **165**: 1287–90.
8. Stovall TG, Solomon SK, Ling FW (1989) Endometrial sampling prior to hysterectomy. *Obstet Gynecol* **73**: 405–9. [erratum appears in *Obstet Gynecol* **74** (1989) 105].
9. Hallez JP, Perino A (1988) Endoscopic intrauterine resection: principles and technique. *Acta Eur Fertil* **19**: 17–21.
10. Rankin L, Steinberg LH (1992) Transcervical resection of the endometrium: a review of 400 consecutive patients. *Br J Obstet Gynaecol* **99**: 911–14.
11. Norwegian Cancer Registry (1987) *Norwegian Cancer Registry Annual Yearbook*. Norwegian Cancer Registry, Oslo.
12. Norris H, Connor M, Kurrmann R (1986) Preinvasive lesions of the endometrium. *Clin Obstet Gynecol* **13**: 725–8.
13. Lewis BV (1994) Guidelines for endometrial ablation. *Br J Obstet Gynaecol* **101**: 470–3.

14. Rybo G (1986) Variation in menstrual blood loss. *Research and Clinical Forums* **4**: 357–74.

15. Fedele L, Bianchi S, Dorta M, Brioschi D, Zanotti F, Vercellini P (1991) Transvaginal ultrasonography versus hysteroscopy in the diagnosis of uterine submucous myomas. *Obstet Gynecol* **77**: 745–8.

16. Goldstein SR (1994) Use of ultrasonohysterography for triage of perimenopausal patients with unexplained uterine bleeding. *Am J Obstet Gynecol* **170**: 565–70.

17. Fraser IS (1990) Hysteroscopy and laparoscopy in women with menorrhagia. *Am J Obstet Gynecol* **162**: 1264–9.

18. Valle RF (1991) Hysteroscopy. *Curr Opin Obstet Gynecol* **3**: 422–6.

19. Altchek A (1992) Management of fibroids. *Curr Opin Obstet Gynecol* **4**: 463–71.

20. Wamsteker K, Emanuel MH, de Kruif JH (1993) Transcervical hysteroscopic resection of submucous fibroids for abnormal uterine bleeding: results regarding the degree of intramural extension. *Obstet Gynecol* **82**: 736–40.

21. Khastgir G, Mascarenhas LJ, Shaxted EJ (1993) The role of transvaginal ultrasonography in pre-operative case selection and post-operative follow up of endometrial resection. *Br J Radiol* 1 **66**: 600–4.

22. Easterday C, Grimes D, Riggs J (1983) Hysterectomy in the United States. *Obstet Gynecol* **62**: 203–12.

23. Rybo G (1966) Menstrual blood loss in relation to parity and menstrual pattern. *Acta Obstet Gynecol Scand Suppl* **45**: 7–27

24. Brooks PG, Serden SP (1992) Endometrial ablation in women with abnormal uterine bleeding aged fifty and over. *J Reprod Med* **37**: 682–4.

25. Sullivan B, Kenney P, Seibel M (1992) Hysteroscopic resection of fibroid with thermal injury to sigmoid. *Obstet Gynecol* **80**: 546–7.

26. Pitroff R (1991) Near fatal uterine perforation during TCRE. *Lancet* **338**: 197–8.

27. Kivnick S, Kanter MH (1992) Bowel injury from rollerball ablation of the endometrium [see comments]. *Obstet Gynecol* **79**: 833–5.

28. Perry C, Daniell JF, Gimpelson RJ (1990) Bowel injury from the Nd:Yag endometrial ablation. *J Gynecol Surg* **6**: 199–203.

29. Indman PD, Brown WW (1992) Uterine surface temperature changes caused by electrosurgical endometrial coagulation. *J Reprod Med* **37**: 667–70.

30. Indman PD, Soderstrom RM (1990) Depth of endometrial coagulation with the urologic resectoscope. *J Reprod Med* **35**: 633–5.

31. Indman PD (1991) High-power Nd:YAG laser ablation of the endometrium. *J Reprod Med* **36**: 501–4.

32. Broadbent JA, Molnar BG, Cooper MJ, Magos AL (1992) Endoscopic management of uterine perforation occurring during endometrial resection. *Br J Obstet Gynaecol* **99**: 1018.

33. Harrison R, Boren J, Robison H (1956) Dilutional hyponatremia shock: another concept of the transurethral prostatic resection reaction. *J Urol* **75**: 95–110.

34. Madsen P, Madsen R (1965) Clinical and experimental evaluation of different irrigation fluids for transurethral surgery. *J Invest Urol* **3**: 122–9.

35. Hoyt H, Goebel J, Shoenbrod J (1958) Types of shock-like reaction during transuretral resection and relation to acute renal failure. *J Urol* **79**: 500–5.

36. Henderson D, Middelton R (1980) Coma from hyponatraemia following transurethral resection of the prostate. *Urology* **15**: 267–71.

37. Shepard RL, Kraus SE, Babayan RK, Siroky MB (1987) The role of ammonia toxicity in the post-transurethral prostatectomy syndrome. *Br J Urol* **60**: 349–51.

38. Perier C, Frey J, Auboyer C *et al.* (1988) Accumulation of glycolic acid and glyoxylic acid in serum in cases of transient hyperglycinemia after transurethral surgery. *Clin Chem* **34**: 1471–3.

39. Goldenberg M, Zolti M, Seidman DS, Bider D, Mashiach S, Etchin A (1994) Transient blood oxygen desaturation, hypercapnia, and coagulopathy after operative hysteroscopy with glycine used as the distending medium. *Am J Obstet Gynecol* **170**: 25–9.

40. Istre O, Skajaa K, Schjoensby AP, Forman A (1992) Changes in serum electrolytes after transcervical resection of endometrium and submucous fibroids with use of glycine 1.5% for uterine irrigation. *Obstet Gynecol* **80**: 218–22.

41. Huxtable RJ (1989) *Taurine and the Oxidative Metabolism of Cystine: Biochemestry of Sulfur.* Plunum Press, New York, pp. 693–734.

42. Istre O, Bjoennes J, Naess R, Hornbaek K, Forman A (1994) Postoperative cerebral oedema after transcervical endometrial resection and uterine irrigation with 1.5% glycine. *Lancet* **344**: 1187–9.

43. MacDonald R, Phipps JH, Singer A (1992) Endometrial ablation: a safe procedure. *Gynaecol Endosc* **1**: 7–9.

44. McCausland VM, Fields GA, McCausland AM, Townsend DE (1993) Tuboovarian abscesses after operative hysteroscopy. *J Reprod Med* **38**: 198–200.

45. Thomas JS Jr, Clark JF (1989) Adenomyosis: a retrospective view. *J Natl Med Assoc* **81**: 969–72.

46. Azziz R (1989) Adenomyosis: current perspectives. *Obstet Gynecol Clin North Am* **16**: 221–35.

47. Vercellini P, Ragni G, Trespidi L, Oldani S, Panazza S, Crosignani PG (1993) Adenomyosis: a deja vu? *Obstet Gynecol Surv* **48**: 789–94.

48. McCausland AM (1992) Hysteroscopic myometrial biopsy: its use in diagnosing adenomyosis and its clinical application. *Am J Obstet Gynecol* **166**: 1619–26.

49. Holm Nielsen P, Nyland MH, Istre O, Maigaard S, Forman A (1993) Acute tissue effects during transcervical endometrial resection. *Gynecol Obstet Invest* **36**: 119–23.

50. Fraser IS (1994) Menorrhagia: a pragmatic approach to the understanding of causes and the need for investigation. *Br J Obstet Gynaecol* **101**: 3–7.

51. Bird C, Mcelin T, Manalo-Estrella P (1972) The elusive adenomyosis of the uterus revised. *Am J Obstet Gynecol* **112**: 583–93.

52. Cooper JM (1992) Hysteroscopic sterilization. *Clin Obstet Gynecol* **35**: 282–98.

53. Istre O, Skajaa K, Holm Nielsen P, Forman A (1993) The second-look appearance of the uterine cavity after resection of the endometrium. *Gynaecol Endosc* **2**: 189–91.

54. Mongelli JM, Evans AJ (1991) Pregnancy after transcervical endometrial resection. *Lancet* **338**: 578–9 (letter).

55. Wood C, Rogers P (1993) A pregnancy after planned partial endometrial resection. *Aust N Z J Obstet Gynaecol* **33**: 316–18.

56. Friedman A, DeFazio J, DeCherney A (1986) Severe obstetric complications after aggressive treatment of Asherman syndrome. *Obstet Gynecol* **67**: 864–7.

57. Hill DJ, Maher PJ (1992) Pregnancy following endometrial ablation. *Gynaecol Endosc* **1**: 47–9.

58. Hill DJ, Maher PJ, Davison GB, Wood C (1992) Haematometra a complication of endometrial ablation. *Aust N Z J Obstet Gynaecol* **32**: 285–6.

59. Jacobs S, Blumenthal N (1994) Endometrial resection follow up: late onset of pain and the effect of depot medroxyprogesterone acetate. *Br J Obstet Gynaecol* **101**: 605–9.

60. Copperman AB, DeCherney AH, Olive DL (1993) A case of endometrial cancer following endometrial ablation for dysfunctional uterine bleeding. *Obstet Gynecol* **82**: 640–2.

61. Granberg S, Wikland M, Karlsson B, Norstrom A, Friberg LG (1991) Endometrial thickness as measured by endovaginal ultrasonography for identifying endometrial abnormality. *Am J Obstet Gynecol* **164**: 47–52.

Chapter 11
Ectopic Pregnancy
J.G. Grudzinskas and A.M. Lower

Introduction

This chapter reviews the advances in diagnostic strategy that have resulted in a greater proportion of women with ectopic pregnancy presenting before tubal rupture, and thus more amenable to conservative and surgical measures. The therapeutic options available, both medical and surgical, are described in detail, together with the problems of tissue extraction and postoperative surveillance.

Diagnostic strategy

Advances in techniques for the diagnosis of ectopic pregnancy, namely simple and sensitive tests for hCG and transvaginal ultrasonography (TVS; Figure 11.1) have permitted the earlier detection of this condition[1]. In women at risk of ectopic pregnancy, it is possible to make the diagnosis before tubal rupture in up to 90% of cases, thus presenting the clinician with a variety of treatment options especially if future fertility is a consideration[2]. However, unless an embryonic heart action is observed outside the uterus (which can be the case in up to 20% of women screened who are at risk of ectopic pregnancy), the definitive diagnosis of ectopic pregnancy is dependent on diagnostic laparoscopy, following which one may consider any one of the surgical treatments discussed in detail below. The extent of surgery performed, i.e. conservative or radical, will be influenced by the woman's desire for future fertility and the condition of the fallopian tube at the time of surgical intervention.

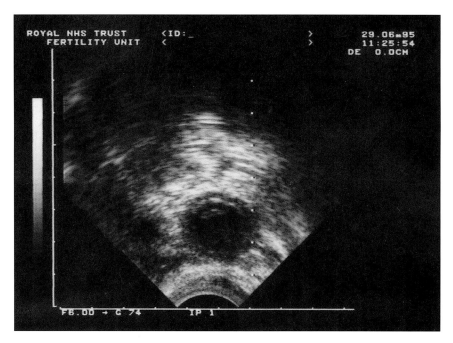

Figure 11.1 *Transvaginal ultrasonogram showing an extrauterine gestational sac.*

Laparoscopy

If ectopic pregnancy is suspected early in modern practice, it is unlikely that the patient will have surgical shock due to haemoperitoneum and require immediate resuscitation and laparotomy. Thus, a diagnostic laparoscopy in women with suspected ectopic pregnancy should be performed with a view to definitive endoscopic treatment in the majority of cases. The general principles of diagnostic laparoscopy (summarized below) are described in detail in Chapter 6, emphasizing the need for good surgical exposure to confirm the diagnosis and assess the site and size of the ectopic pregnancy and the condition of the affected tube, the contralateral tube, ovaries and other pelvic organs. The appropriate surgical treatment, reflecting the needs of the patient, will be influenced by the patient's wishes for future fertility, her general circulatory condition, the site and size of the ectopic pregnancy, the condition of the affected tube and the contralateral tube, and whether the affected tube has been the site of ectopic pregnancy previously.

Aims of diagnostic laparoscopy for ectopic pregnancy

- Good surgical exposure
- Confirmation of the diagnosis
- Assessment of the size and site of ectopic pregnancy
- Assessment of the condition of the affected tube
- Assessment of the condition of the contralateral tube
- Assessment of the condition of the ovaries and other pelvic organs

---

Therapeutic options

Expectant management

Although surgery is the mainstay of treatment, expectant treatment with spontaneous resolution of tubal pregnancy can be considered in women with unruptured ectopic pregnancy and low and declining serum hCG levels (<2000 IU/l) who can comply with the demands of frequent follow-up visits. Up to 20% of women with ectopic pregnancy may satisfy these criteria, and about half of them will have uneventful and safe spontaneous resolution of their ectopic pregnancy[3].

Medical management (Figure 11.2)

Systemic medical treatment by the intravenous, intramuscular or intratubal administration of methotrexate is also effective if the tubal

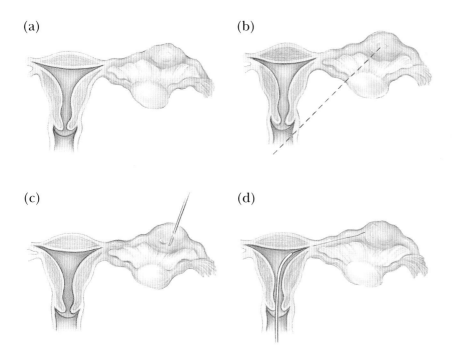

Figure 11.2 *Medical management of ectopic pregnancy: (a) systemic, b) transvaginal injection, (c) local transabdominal or laparoscopic injection, (d) transcervical.*

mass is small (<2 cm) and serum hCG levels low (<2000 IU/l)[2]. Advocates of this technique cite technical simplicity and shorter operating time as advantages.

Local medical treatment at diagnostic videolaparoscopy with the injection of agents such as methotrexate, prostaglandin F_{2a} or glucose can be performed in early ectopic pregnancy[4], successfully treating the condition in 90% of women. A novel approach using the transcervical route by cannulation of the fallopian tube by touch or microendoscopic techniques has also been described[5].

Surgical management (Figure 11.3)

Thorough lavage and aspiration of any blood with a good-quality suction irrigation device will permit good exposure of the ectopic pregnancy, demonstrating tubal abortion, an intact ectopic pregnancy or a ruptured ectopic pregnancy.

Figure 11.3 *Surgical management of ectopic pregnancy: (a) salpingectomy, (b) segmental excision, (c) linear salpingostomy.*

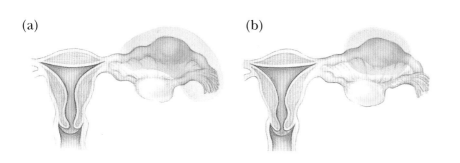
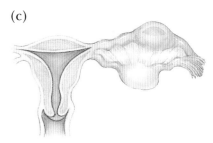

Linear salpingostomy

Linear salpingostomy (Figure 11.4) is the treatment of choice for the intact relatively undamaged tube, especially in women desirous of future fertility. It is ideal for the majority of ectopic pregnancies located in the ampulla. The tube is held steady with grasping forceps. Some surgeons inject a vasoconstrictor (1.5–2 ml of dilute vasopressin under the serosa of the mesosalpinx) to assist with haemostasis. A linear incision along the antimesosalpingeal border of the affected tube is made by diathermy needle electrode, laser or scissors introduced through the third portal. If diathermy is used, the fallopian tube should be held against the fundus of the uterus so that it acts as a broad-based return path for the diathermy energy to the ground electrode. This can be facilitated if the uterus is held in retroversion. The incision is commenced beside the gestation sac distal to the uterus and extended towards the uterus until gestational tissues are encountered and begin to extrude. Compression of the tube will facilitate extrusion of the tissue. Tubal tissue will tear easily, causing bleeding, and should not be grasped. Once gestational tissues are protruding from the tube, aquadissection and suction can be used to efficiently remove the ectopic pregnancy.

The tubal lumen and ectopic pregnancy site should be lavaged and carefully inspected to ensure that complete removal has occurred and to identify bleeding, which can be thermocoagulated. The salpingostomy incision is left open to heal satisfactorily, resulting in tubal patency in the majority of women.

Segmental excision

This is the procedure of choice for ectopic pregnancy in the tubal isthmus, but is also used if the ectopic pregnancy is >3 cm in diameter

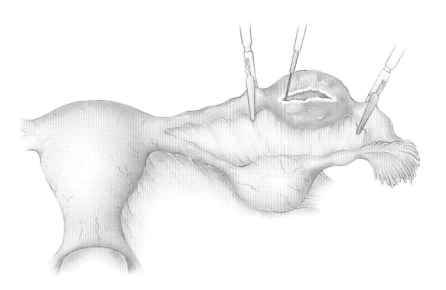

Figure 11.4 *Linear salpingostomy.*

and in the proximal ampulla[6]. Segmental incision (Figure 11.5) may be performed using suturing techniques by ligating the tube proximal and distal to the ectopic pregnancy with 3/0 or 4/0 Vicryl (Ethicon, Edinburgh, UK) or PDS (Ethicon) sutures. The ectopic pregnancy is then further ligated and removed by transection of the adjacent mesosalpinx. This procedure is time consuming by the videolaparoscopic approach, so electrosurgery using monopolar or bipolar techniques is more frequently performed.

Salpingectomy

This is the method of choice where the fallopian tube is obviously damaged by pre-existing disease. Most operators prefer an electrosurgical technique (monopolar or bipolar) similar to the method used for segmental excision of the tube. Sutures such as Endoloop (Ethicon) or Surgitie (Auto Suture, Ascot, UK) may also be used.

The affected tube is grasped together with the mesosalpinx, electrocoagulated and cut at the uterotubal junction (Figure 11.6), thus occluding the blood supply to the tube. The tubo-ovarian ligament is grasped, diathermied and divided. The mesosalpinx is then electrocoagulated and cut, excising the tube.

Pre-tied surgical slip knots such as the Endoloop or Surgitie can be used to secure haemostasis of vascular pedicles; the mesosalpinx is particularly suited to this technique. A grasping forceps is passed through the loop and the portion of the tube to be excised is drawn through the loop. The loop is then cinched down onto the mesosalpinx using the integral knot pusher. For security, three loops are usually applied to highly vascular structures such as the mesosalpinx.

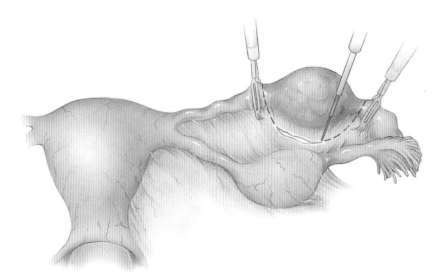

Figure 11.5 *Segmental excision.*

Figure 11.6 *Salpingectomy.*

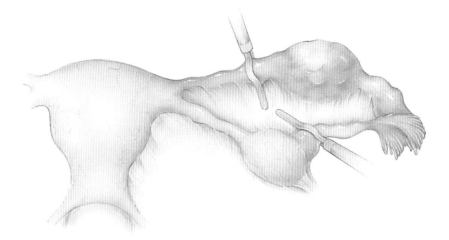

Tissue extraction

The techniques of removing tissues from the abdomen are described in detail elsewhere. Typically, tissues may be removed through an 11 mm cannula, the procedure being viewed through another port. Repeated morcellation of the specimen will facilitate removal without necessitating an increase in the size of existing incisions. Larger specimens are removed through a posterior colpotomy.

Postoperative care

Typically, women treated for unruptured ectopic pregnancy may be discharged within 12–24 h of the procedure. If there is concern about residual trophoblastic tissue, weekly serial β-hCG determinations should be performed.

Advantages of laparoscopic management of ectopic pregnancy

- Lower cost
- Less morbidity
- Shorter convalescence
- Better cosmetic result
- Speedier return to full activity

Summary

Early diagnosis of ectopic pregnancy leads to the diagnosis being made prior to rupture of the fallopian tube, the woman thus being more amenable to laparoscopic surgery. The extent of laparoscopic surgery required will be influenced by the woman's choice to retain her fertility as well as size of the gestation sac, whether tubal rupture has occurred, the state of the contra-lateral tube and the presence of any other pelvic pathology. Laparoscopic treatment is still possible and desirable even if tubal rupture has occurred and a haemoperitoneum is present. The availability of laparoscopic surgical expertise and equipment should be the major factors in deciding whether to perform endoscopic surgery. Surgery will include salpingostomy, partial or total salpingectomy. It is also possible to injection cytotoxic drugs, e.g. methotrexate, under direct vision if appropriate. The duration of hospitalization and convalescence is greatly reduced.

References

1. Stabile I, Grudzinskas JG (1995) Ectopic pregnancy: What's new? In: Studd JW (ed.) Progress in Obstetrics and Gynaecology. Churchill Livingston, London, p.11.
2. Balasch J, Barri PN (1994) Treatment of ectopic pregnancy: the new gynaecological dilemma. *Hum Reprod* **9**: 547–58.
3. Carson SA, Buster JE (1993) Ectopic pregnancy. *N Engl J Med* **329**: 1174–81.
4. Lindblom B (1994) Non-surgical approaches in ectopic pregnancy: systemic medical treatment of local injection therapy? In: Grudzinskas JG, Chard T, Djahanbakhch O (eds) Fallopian Tube: Basic Science and Clinical Aspects. London, Springer-Verlag, pp. 271–7.
5. Risquez A (1994) Transcervical tubal cannulation and ectopic pregnancy. In: Grudzinskas JG, Chard T, Djahanbakhch O (eds) Fallopian Tube: Basic Science and Clinical Aspects. Springer-Verlag, pp. 279–93.
6. Gomel V (1994) Management of tubal pregnancy: transabdominal. In: Grudzinskas JG, Chard T, Djahanbakhch O (eds) Fallopian Tube: Basic Science and Clinical Aspects. Springer-Verlag, pp. 255–69.

Chapter 12
Reproductive Surgery
A.M. Lower and C.J.G. Sutton

Introduction

This chapter describes the surgical procedures available to the reproductive surgeon. The procedures are outlined and, where possible, the results of trials to assess their effectiveness are presented. There is a lack of adequately controlled prospective trials to conclusively prove the benefit of the endoscopic approach over the open procedure, and in many cases open procedures have not been adequately justified. The difficulty with such trials lies in the multifactorial nature of infertility and the difficulty in identifying suitable end-points and outcomes for studies. Infertility is relative, and few conditions are associated with absolute infertility, so that treatment-independent pregnancies may cloud the results of trials.

Advantages of endoscopic surgery

Endoscopic surgery for infertility is a particularly attractive alternative to open surgery for a number of reasons. Most women presenting with subfertility patients are in regular employment and, especially where there is no guarantee of success, prefer to return to work as quickly as possible after surgical intervention. The minimal-access approach assists this. It may also allow sexual intercourse to occur sooner after surgery than with a painful Pfannenstiel incision, thus exposing the woman to an earlier chance of conception. Practical considerations aside, endoscopic surgery also embraces the principles of microsurgery, listed below. In addition, the laparoscopic approach is associated with less risk of infection and less postoperative adhesion formation.

Principles of microsurgery

- Adequate exposure
- Magnification
- Minimal tissue handling
- Strict attention to haemostasis
- Prevention of tissue desiccation

Tubal surgery

Adhesiolysis

Overall, surgery for peritubal adhesions appears to be associated with poor results. This is largely due to poor patient selection. Most authors agree that, if surgery is restricted to patients with less extensive disease, worthwhile pregnancy rates can be obtained. Where there is more extensive disease or an additional male infertility factor, women should be offered *in vitro* fertilization with embryo transfer (IVF-ET). Figure 12.1 shows the cumulative conception rates for open tubal surgery from a number of studies reviewed by Hull[1].

Tulandi *et al.*[2] compared the fertility rates in 69 women receiving open tubal surgery and 78 managed expectantly. There was no significant difference in the degree of adhesions between the two groups. The cumulative pregnancy rates using life-table analysis, at 12 and 24 months' follow-up, respectively, were 32% and 45% in the treated group and 11% and 16% in the non-treated group, showing a clear benefit of treatment.

Laparoscopic salpingo-ovariolysis is particularly suitable for patients with apparently normal fallopian tubes at hysterosalpingoscopy, but in whom tubal motility and ovum retrieval may be hampered by the presence of external adhesions caused by previous surgery or infection, for example complicated acute appendicitis.

Donnez, who was a practising microsurgeon before he took up laser laparoscopic surgery, reported 108 (58%) viable pregnancies in 186 patients for stage 1 disease[3]. Similar results were obtained by MacDonald and Sutton with 34 of 56 women (61%) becoming

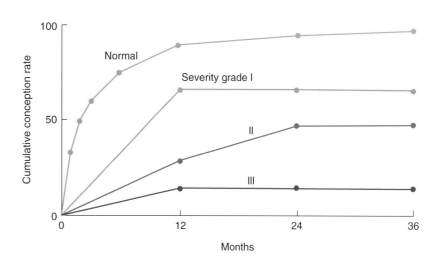

Figure 12.1 *Cumulative conception rates for open tubal surgery related to disease grading compared with normal. The most severe cases (grade IV) were not operated on. (From ref.1).*

pregnant, the majority within six cycles following laser laparoscopic adhesiolysis. In neither series were any ectopic pregnancies reported.

Similar success rates have been reported by laparoscopic surgeons using scissors, with or without electrosurgery[4–6], but these series all have reported ectopic rates between 5 and 8%.

Surgical technique

This is a truly minimal-access procedure, and most procedures can be completed using only two 5 mm accessory ports (one in each iliac fossa) because no tissue needs to be removed. Sometimes a third 5 mm port is required, placed suprapubically.

The instruments used are atraumatic grasping forceps (which may be used to grasp the bowel or tube to put the adhesions on stretch), a cutting instrument (usually scissors, electrocautery needle electrode or surgical laser) and, most importantly, a good suction/irrigation probe. An experienced assistant is essential because the technique requires the surgeon to use both hands at once to tease apart adhesions. One of the grasping forceps is then given to the assistant so that the adhesions may be kept on stretch while being cut or vaporized. Care must be exercised in the use of electrocautery close to the bowel or on the pelvic sidewall over the ureter (see Chapter 5).

A number of different endoscopic techniques have been described for adhesiolysis, including the use of scissors (with and without electrocautery), lasers (carbon dioxide, Nd-YAG, KTP or diode) and fine needle diathermy. The results appear to be similar, whatever method is used (Table 12.1).

Some authors have claimed that treatment by competent microsurgery gives better results than multiple cycles of IVF in selected patients[7]. This may no longer be true as success rates with IVF improve. What is clear is that careful patient selection, thorough investigation to reach an accurate diagnosis, and appropriate tailoring of treatment to individuals is the gold standard for which we should all be aiming.

Table 12.1 *Outcome after laparoscopic adhesiolysis using different surgical methods*

Author	Year	Surgical method	N	Follow-up (years)	Pregnancy rate (%)
Gomel[5]	1983	Scissors	92	1	67.4
Fayez	1983	Scissors	50	2	60
Mettler et al.[14]	1979	Diathermy	44	1–6	29.5
Bruhat et al.[6]	1983	Diathermy	93	1	59.1
Donnez and Nisolle[3]	1989	Laser	186	1.5	58
Sutton	1992	Laser	56	1–7	61.7

Laser surgery

Lasers offer safer, more precise division and vaporization. A confusing range of lasers is available. Essentially they achieve their effect either by the direct action of optically transmitted laser energy, as in the carbon dioxide laser, or by the effect of laser energy delivered by a quartz fibre to either a moulded tip or a replaceable crystal tip which becomes heated, as in the Nd-YAG, KTP and diode lasers.

The carbon dioxide laser offers some advantages over other operative techniques for endometriosis and adhesions but, in spite of the continuing development of new instrumentation, there are still problems with the system. The technique needs specialized equipment requiring ongoing biomedical maintenance and specialized technical care in the operating room. Problems such as the intraperitoneal accumulation of smoke, gas leakage, and difficulty with maintenance of proper beam alignment still occur. In spite of these problems the system allows precise bloodless destruction of diseased tissue and eliminates the risks of cautery. In the hands of an experienced laparoscopist, it appears safe and effective in the vaporization of endometriotic lesions, uterosacral neurectomy, adhesiolysis and salpingostomy. The outcome of carefully planned further investigations by well trained and experienced laparoscopists is awaited.

The diode, Nd-YAG, KTP and other fibre delivery systems all work in a similar fashion: the laser energy is used to achieve heating of the fibre tip. This has a low specific heat capacity and thus cools and heats up very quickly, acting as a point source of heat. These instruments have advantages over surgical diathermy in that there is no return current path to be considered. Some surgeons also prefer the physical contact and tactile feedback offered by fibre delivery systems over carbon dioxide systems. The fibre systems are also easier to use because the transmission through tissue is very much less than with carbon dioxide lasers, and a backstop does not need to be employed. The laser with which one of the authors (AML) has most experience is shown in Figure 12.2. The attractive features of this instrument are its small size, rugged solid-state construction and portability.

At present, lasers have been used in an unsophisticated fashion, using their immense power to vaporize tissue. The differential absorption of energy of different wavelengths has not been extensively explored. Carbon dioxide laser energy is readily absorbed by water and hence vaporizes most cells in an indiscriminate fashion. Energy of other wavelengths, such as those produced by diode, argon, Nd-YAG, KTP, krypton, xenon, copper and gold vapour lasers, has different properties of penetration, absorption, reflection and heat dissipation. Photodynamic therapy using photosensitizers and fluorescing agents may lead to new therapeutic possibilities. This has already been shown to be a promising treatment of experimentally induced endometriosis in rabbits[8].

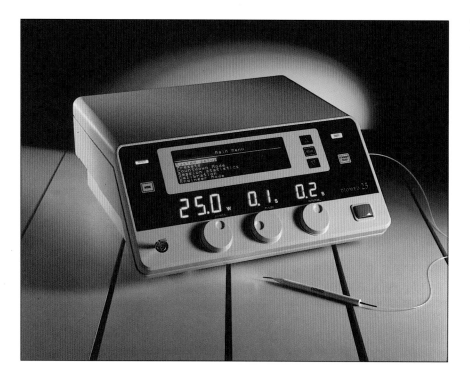

Figure 12.2 *The Diomed 25 surgical diode laser.*

Other possible therapeutic applications of lasers include endoscopic holography, in which a krypton ion laser is attached to a contact endoscope allowing three-dimensional holography of the endosalpinx, endometrium or internal surface of an ovarian cyst. Holographic interferometry uses a signal from a double-pulsed ruby laser to measure and visualize dynamic events such as ciliary beating of the endosalpinx, providing a dynamic assessment of tubal function[9].

Neosalpingostomy and fimbrioplasty

Tubal surgery is less successful when the tubes are not patent. In a retrospective review of the results of open microsurgical salpingostomy for bilateral distal tubal blockage at the Hammersmith Hospital between 1971 and 1988, 39% of almost 100 women with stage I disease conceived after primary salpingostomy and 25% after repeat salpingostomy[7]. Over half the women having a term pregnancy subsequently had a second infant. Other authors have reported similar figures[10–12]. Proper selection of patients, competent microsurgical technique and adequate follow-up appear to be crucial to success. Success rates are adversely affected by previous surgery, thick-walled hydrosalpinges and deciliation of the fallopian tube mucosa. More extensive disease has a lower success rate and higher ectopic rate.

There are no useful trials comparing laparoscopic treatment with open surgery directly; however, Donnez has published two similar studies[3,11] reporting the outcome after conventional open microsurgery in 1986 and after laparoscopic adhesiolysis using the carbon dioxide laser in 1989. The term pregnancy rate after fimbrioplasty for occlusion of degree I and salpingostomy for occlusion of degree II was more than 50% following open surgery. In the later, laparoscopic series 57% of women conceived during the 18 month follow-up period.

Surgical technique

It is usually necessary to perform a salpingolysis, as described above, to display the tube adequately. Methylene blue is then injected into the uterus through the cervix to confirm that there is no cornual blockage and to distend the tubes. Bipolar (concurrent proximal and distal) disease has a particularly poor prognosis and should not be treated surgically. Once the tubes have been distended, the thinnest part of the adhesions overlying the fimbriated end of the tube is identified and incised in a classic terminal salpingostomy. This incision is then extended and an assessment made of the mucosa and fimbrial epithelium of the tube. Low-power laser energy or electrocautery can be used to cause the mildest blanching and shrinkage of the serosa of the tube a few millimetres from the neosalpingostomy, which will cause flowering out of the tube and prevent it from closing over again (Figure 12.3).

(a)

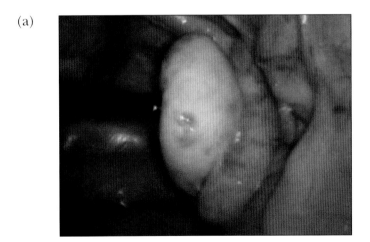

(b)

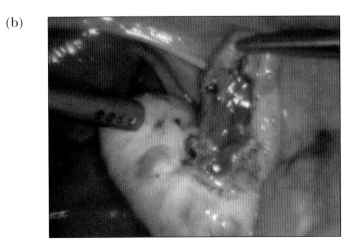

Figure 12.3 *(a) Preoperative and (b) postoperative neosalpingostomy technique.*

As with laparoscopic adhesiolysis, the results of a variety of surgical methods have been reported[13-16] (Table 12.2). The success rates appear to be similar and largely independent of the method used.

It is reasonable to conclude from the foregoing that the results of tubal surgery are largely similar following laparoscopic and open surgery. The surgical method employed appears to be less important than the extent of the disease, and women with patent tubes are more likely to conceive after surgery than those with hydrosalpinges. Further prospective studies are required to determine the place of surgical management rather than assisted conception techniques in the treatment of infertility.

Tubal reanastomosis

There are no trials comparing laparoscopic tubal reanastomosis with open surgery. As yet there are only a few case reports of successful laparoscopic tubal reanastomosis[17-19]. The main difficulty appears to lie in accurate tissue apposition and the time-consuming practice of intracorporeal suturing techniques. The time taken to complete the anastomosis is greater in laparoscopic procedures, and some authorities have claimed that the results are inferior. The use of tissue glues and welding techniques may go some way to overcoming these difficulties. Further prospective evaluation is required.

Adnexal surgery

Endometriosis

The exact mechanism by which endometriosis causes infertility is not clear; however, this condition has been shown to be associated with marked subfertility[1]. Figure 12.4 shows the cumulative pregnancy curves for minor, moderate and severe grades of untreated endometriosis.

Table 12.2 *Outcome after laparoscopic neosalpingostomy using different surgical methods*

Author	Year	Surgical method	N	Follow-up (years)	Pregnancy rate (%)
Gomel[4]	1983	Scissors	9	1	44.4
Mettler et al.[13]	1979	Scissors	36	1–6	26
Fayez	1983	Scissors	19	2	10
Daniell and Herbert[16]	1984	Carbon dioxide laser	21	1–1.5	24
Donnez and Nisolle[3]	1989	Carbon dioxide laser	25	1.5	20
Dubuisson et al.[15]	1990	Combined	34	1.5	32.4

Figure 12.4 *Cumulative conception rates (percentages of couples conceiving) in the normal population and in untreated endometriosis of different degrees of severity.*

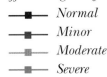

—■— *Normal*
—■— *Minor*
—■— *Moderate*
—■— *Severe*

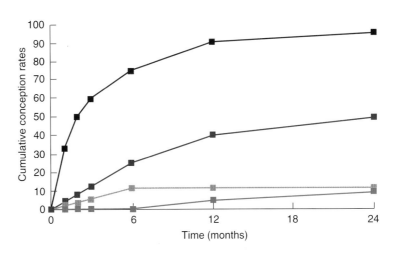

Nowroozi and colleagues reported a randomized prospective trial to determine whether laparoscopic treatment of mild endometriosis was associated with an improved pregnancy rate[20]. One hundred and twenty-three women were randomly allocated to either treatment or no treatment groups. All other infertility factors were meticulously corrected before laparoscopic treatment, and patients were allowed at least eight 'normal' cycles before their endometriosis was treated. Of 69 patients receiving laparoscopic fulguration of endometriotic implants, 42 (61%) achieved a pregnancy within eight cycles following treatment. Only 10 of 54 patients from the control group (19%) conceived in the same time period.

Sutton and colleagues have recently presented the interim findings of the Guildford Birthright Study, a double-blind randomized prospective study comparing the outcome of patients with endometriosis stages I–III (revised American Fertility Society (rAFS) staging) treated by laser or expectant management. Patients in the expectant arm underwent hydrotubation and aspiration of accumulated peritoneal fluid from the cul-de-sac. After 1 year of follow-up, seven of 14 (50%) in the laser arm and three of 13 (23%) in the expectant arm became pregnant[21].

By comparison, no benefit in terms of improved pregnancy rate was demonstrated with hormonal treatment[20]. The relation between asymptomatic endometriosis and infertility was investigated in a randomized double-blind placebo-controlled trial of the impact of treating the endometriosis with gestrinone. The 12 month cumulative conception rate in patients treated with gestrinone was 25% (five of 20) and in those given placebo 24% (four of 17). These patients were then divided into those in whom no visible endometriosis was present at second laparoscopy and those in whom residual disease was present, and the 12 month cumulative conception rates were 25% (four of 16) and 30% (six of 20), respectively. None of these rates differed significantly, and they compared with a rate of 23% (six of 26) in a control group of patients with unexplained infertility. Patients in whom the disease was eliminated did not return to normal fertility, although all other causes of infertility were excluded. This study failed to show any impact of treatment or the absence or presence of asymptomatic endometriosis on future fertility.

Interestingly, the prognosis for fertility appears to be unrelated to severity of disease or method of treatment (Table 12.3)[22].

Surgical technique

The aim of surgical treatment is to remove all visible endometriotic deposits. This can be done with laser, diathermy or recently introduced instruments such as the argon beam coagulator and harmonic scalpel. Each of these achieves satisfactory vaporization, although the laser is the most precise and causes least collateral damage.

Peritoneal endometriosis

Typical appearances are shown in Figure 12.5. These range from classical 'powder-burn' deposits to more subtle changes such as abnormal vascular changes and scarring from old lesions. The carbon dioxide laser is particularly suited to dealing with these types of lesion. Sharplan (Tel-Aviv, Israel) have developed the Swiftlase system, which defocuses the beam and diffuses it over the surface to vaporize a larger area of tissue. The technique of hydrodissection is often used: a small window is cut in the peritoneum and water injected behind so that the peritoneum is gently separated from the underlying tissue. The ready absorption of carbon dioxide laser energy by water provides protection from inadvertent damage, and the peritoneum can be vaporized quickly and safely, ensuring adequate clearance of all endometriotic tissue.

The moulded-tip delivery fibres used with the diode laser can be employed in a similar fashion. A 1 mm diameter orb-tipped fibre is used to vaporize classic powder-burn lesions. Penetration is limited to 400 μm, and in vitro studies have shown collateral to be limited to less than 200 μm, ensuring safe utilization, especially on the pelvic sidewall

	Severity of endometriosis			
	Minimal	Mild	Moderate	Severe
Electrocautery	28/44	110/210	24/67	4/8
	64%	52%	36%	50%
Carbon dioxide laser	329/553	230/397	94/162	37/58
	59%	58%	58%	64%

Table 12.3 *Prognosis for fertility after surgery for varying severity of endometriosis*

Figure 12.5 *Peritoneal endometriosis.*

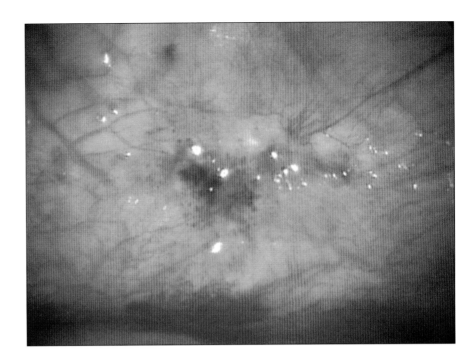

overlying important structures such as the ureter and major vessels. Diathermy can be used, but its action is less precise than that of a laser.

Ovarian endometriomata

There are two schools of thought as to the best management of ovarian endometriomata. One (favoured by one of the authors: CJGS) recommends fenestration of the chocolate cyst, thorough irrigation and inspection of the cyst cavity, and laser ablation of the internal surface of the capsule using a KTP laser. Others favour drainage of the cyst and stripping the capsule from the normal ovarian tissue. The other author (AML) favours the latter approach where possible, although when the capsule does not strip away easily, which is sometimes the case after prolonged treatment with GnRH analogues or in the presence of extensive adhesions, laser ablation of the internal surface of the capsule has been employed with good effect.

Sutton has recently reported his experience with large endometriomata (between 3 and 18 cm in diameter) during the past 10 years. The mean rAFS score was 45 and the mean duration of infertility was 53 months. Of the 42 women actively trying to conceive, 24 (57%) were successful, usually within 8 months of surgery. In all, 52 of 71 (73%) had resolution of pain[23].

Polycystic ovarian syndrome

Ovarian drilling

The majority of women with polycystic ovarian syndrome (PCO) will respond to simple medical measures: approximately 60% will conceive on clomiphene citrate alone. The remainder represent a more challenging group. Gonadotrophin therapy will be successful in some, but this requires careful monitoring and may lead to ovarian hyperstimulation and the risk of multiple pregnancy. Surgical management of this condition has previously included wedge resection of the ovaries, now largely abandoned because of the frequent occurrence of adhesions between the ovaries and fallopian tubes.

Recently, the creation of multiple lesions in the ovarian capsule using either diathermy or laser has been described as an alternative[23]. The results of initial trials have been most encouraging[24]. In a study of 50 women with clomiphene-resistant PCO, 43 women (86%) ovulated following ovarian diathermy; the mean (SD) time to ovulation was 23 (6.2) days. Three non-responders ovulated following antioestrogen treatment to which they were previously resistant. Thirty-three women have conceived 58 pregnancies. The exact mechanism by which this alters the underlying metabolic defect is not clear. However, recent data suggest that the effect is obtained even if surgery is restricted to one ovary (Balen, personal communication).

The long-term effect of ovarian drilling is not yet certain. Concern has been expressed that destruction of ovarian tissue by ovarian drilling may lead to premature menopause but, in one study, women who had undergone wedge resection of the ovaries for PCO between 22 and 33 years previously were shown to have reached the menopause at a similar age to age-matched controls[25]. There is an improvement in the metabolic disturbance; however, most patients seem to relapse between 2 and 3 years after treatment.

At present this surgery should be restricted to women who fail to respond to clomiphene citrate. There may be a place for ovarian drilling in women with PCO before ovarian stimulation for IVF. Anecdotal experience suggests that the brittle response characteristic in these women, often resulting in ovarian hyperstimulation syndrome, may be avoided following ovarian drainage. This work needs further clarification and confirmation.

Surgical technique

A number of lesions are created on the surface of the ovary using either diathermy or laser. If diathermy is used, great care must be exercised to ensure that the return current passes through the pelvic sidewall or the uterus by holding the ovary against the uterine fundus or sidewall while the diathermy energy is applied. If the return current is allowed to pass down the ovarian pedicle the ovarian vein may be thrombosed and the ovary lost in consequence.

Using diathermy, four or five lesions 5 mm in diameter and up to 8 mm in depth are created on the surface of each ovary. More lesions are required with lasers because the amount of ovarian tissue damaged is less. The ovary is then cooled using irrigating fluid.

Safety point

The ovary must be held in contact with the fundus of the uterus to avoid the passage of return current through the ovarian vein.

Uterine surgery

Hysteroscopic resection of septa

Abnormalities of the uterine cavity may affect fertility by inhibiting implantation or causing early miscarriage. Gaucherand *et al.*[26] evaluated the obstetric and perinatal implications of the septate uterus. In a retrospective study of 203 pregnancies in 78 women with untreated septate uterus, they found that the fetal loss rate during the first two trimesters was 47%, prematurity 17% and only 89 children survived (i.e. the overall perinatal mortality rate was 16.8% when pregnancy exceeded 24 weeks). Subsequently, 25 women underwent surgical treatment of the septum. In this group, the proportion of pregnancies proceeding beyond 24 weeks' gestation increased from 13 to 90%, and infant survival increased from 4 to 88%.

Surgical technique

It is essential that the surgeon is thoroughly familiar with diagnostic hysteroscopy and capable of recognizing abnormal anatomy. The most commonly used instruments include a standard operating hysteroscope with a two-way irrigation channel and diathermy loop or a smaller diameter diagnostic hysteroscope with a 5 Fr instrument channel through which can be introduced semi-rigid biopsy forceps, scissors, microdiathermy instruments or a laser fibre (Figures 12.6–12.7). These instruments are used under video control to dissect or vaporize the septum or adhesions[27–29]. The results of each seem to be comparable, and operator experience and familiarity is the important factor. Thorough preoperative assessment is essential and transvaginal ultrasonography and hysterosalpingography are mandatory. It is prudent to perform a control laparoscopy to minimize the risk of uterine perforation and to differentiate between septate and bicornuate uterus. Typical hysteroscopic appearance of a uterine septum are shown in Figure 12.8.

The hysteroscopic approach has also been described in the treatment of intrauterine adhesions (Asherman's syndrome) associated with infertility (Figure 12.9). No large studies or prospective data are available for this relatively uncommon condition. In severe cases it can be difficult to visualize the tubal ostia, which generally serve as landmarks when performing intrauterine dissection. In such cases transvesical or transrectal ultrasound guidance can be very useful in ensuring that the correct plane is being developed within the uterus.

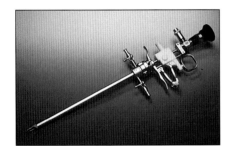

Figure 12.6 *Olympus continuous flow resectoscope (courtesy of KeyMed (Medical & Industrial Equipment) Ltd, Southend-on-Sea, UK).*

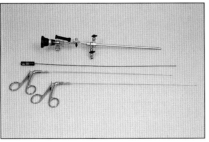

Figure 12.7 *Olympus continuous flow hysteroscope with 5 Fr instrument channel (courtesy of KeyMed (Medical & Industrial Equipment) Ltd, Southend-on-Sea, UK).*

Myomectomy

It has been suggested that uterine fibroids are associated with recurrent miscarriage, implantation failure and infertility. The evidence, in the form of randomized prospective trials, is lacking; however, it is generally agreed that where the fibroid significantly distorts the uterine cavity, or causes symptoms such as menorrhagia, pain or urinary and bowel symptoms due to local pressure effects, surgical treatment should be considered.

Excision of uterine fibroids at laparotomy has been described and reviewed by a number of authors[30-32], reporting successful pregnancy rates of between 40 and 65%. However, there is a significant morbidity with, in many cases, substantial blood loss and prolonged recovery.

Endoscopic treatment has been advocated using either the hysteroscopic approach or laparoscopy, depending on the site of the fibroid. A variety of surgical methods have been described, including electrocautery and carbon dioxide, Nd-YAG, argon and KTP lasers. Their use has been fully described elsewhere[33].

There are limited reports of pregnancy rates following surgery for fibroids. Smith and Uhlir[34] report a series of 64 myomectomies performed at open surgery. Although infertility was not the primary indication in any case, 40% of those attempting to conceive after surgery achieved a successful pregnancy. Loffer[35] reports successful conception in seven of 12 women (58%) attempting to conceive after hysteroscopic resection of fibroids. Further studies are required before any reasonable conclusions can be drawn concerning the benefits of surgery in women with fibroids.

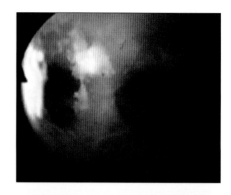

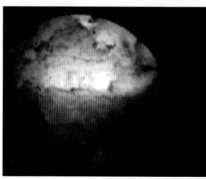

Figure 12.8 *Typical hysteroscopic appearance of a uterine septum. (a) Preoperative and (b) post resection views.*

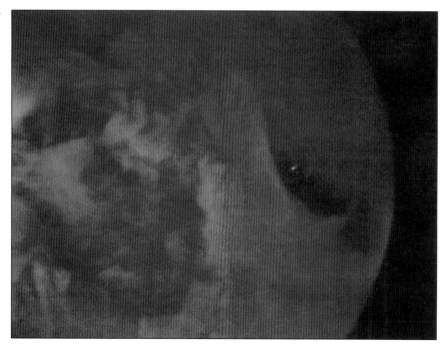

Figure 12.9 *Asherman's syndrome.*

LUNA

Laparoscopic uterine nerve ablation (LUNA) is a useful manoeuvre in women suffering from dysmenorrhoea caused by endometriosis or adenomyosis who wish to preserve their reproductive potential. This technique has been described using carbon dioxide laser, Nd-YAG laser and electrocautery. A success rate of 73% has been claimed in terms of relief of pain following this procedure in women with primary dysmenorrhoea and 86% in those with endometriosis[36]. In a prospective randomized trial of 21 women with persistent, severe or incapacitating dysmenorrhoea with no demonstrable pelvic pathology which was resistant to non-steroidal anti-inflammatory drugs, nine of 11 patients (82%) reported relief of symptoms after LUNA, whereas none in the control group experienced any relief[37]. The effect of LUNA on fertility is unclear, although it may enable the uterus to be preserved in cases of incapacitating dysmenorrhoea where the only alternative treatment would have been hysterectomy.

Summary

In the hands of an experienced laparoscopist, it appears that safe and effective vaporization of endometriotic lesions, uterosacral nerve ablation, adhesiolysis and salpingostomy may be adequately performed with results broadly comparable to those of open procedures. Operative hysteroscopy may have a place in the management of intrauterine adhesions, fibroids and Mullerian duct abnormalities.

As more surgeons are trained in these challenging techniques, it is likely that interest will be renewed in the surgical treatment of infertility, which is currently partially eclipsed by IVF and related treatments.

References

1. Hull MGR (1994). In: Templeton AA, Drife JO (eds) Infertilty. Springer-Verlag, London, pp.33-62.
2. Tulandi T, Collins JA, Burrows E, Jarrell JF, McInnes RA, Wrixon W (1990). Treatment-dependent and treatment-independent pregnancy among women with periadnexal adhesions. *Am J Obstet Gynecol* **162**: 354-7.
3. Donnez J, Nisolle M (1989) CO_2 laser laparoscopic surgery: adhesiolysis, salpingostomy, laser uterine nerve ablation and tubal pregnancy. *Baillieres Clin Obstet Gynaecol* **3**: 525-43.
4. Gomel V (1983). Salpingo-ovariolysis by laparoscopy in infertility. *Fertil Steril* **40**: 607-11.
5. Bruhat MA, Mage G, Manhes H, Soualhat C, Ropert JF, Pouly JL (1983). Laparoscopy procedures to promote fertiltity, ovariolyosis and salpingolysis: results of 93 selected cases. *Acta Eur Fertil* **14**; 113-15.
6. Reich H, McGlynn F (1986). Treatment of ovarian endometriosis using laparoscopic surgical techniques. *J Reprod Med* **31**: 577-84.
7. Winston RM, Margara RA (1991). Microsurgical salpingostomy is not an obsolete procedure. *Br J Obstet Gynaecol* **98**: 637-42.

8. Keye WR (1992) In: Sutton CJG (ed.) Lasers in Gynaecology. Chapman & Hall, London, pp.257-67.
9. Sutton CJG (1991). What can we expect from the surgical management of endometriosis ? *Br J Clin Pract Symp Suppl* **72**: 33-42.
10. Mage G, Bruhat MA (1983). Pregancy following salpingostomy: comparison between CO_2 laser and electrosurgery procedures. *Fertil Steril* **40**: 472-5.
11. Donnez J, Casanas-Roux F (1986). Prognostic factors of fimbrial microsurgery. *Fertil Steril* **46**: 200-4.
12. Mage G, Pouly JL, Bouquet de Joliniere J, Chabrand S, Bruhat MA (1984). Distal tubal obstructions: microsurgery or *in vitro* fertilisation. *J Gynecol Obstet Biol Reprod* **13**: 933-7.
13. Mettler L, Giesel H, Semm K (1979). Treatment of female infertility due to tubal obstruction by operative laparoscopy. *Fertil Steril* **32**: 384-8.
14. Donnez J, Casanas-Roux F (1986). Prognostc factors influencing the pregnancy rate after microsurgical cornual anastomosis. *Fertil Steril* **32**: 1089-92.
15. Dubuisson JB, Bouquet de Joliniere J, Aubriot FX, Darai E, Foulot H (1990). Terminal tuboplasties by laparoscopy: 65 consecutive cases. *Fertil Steril* **54**: 401-3.
16. Daniell JF, Herbert CM (1984). Laparoscopic salpingostomy using the CO_2 laser. *Fertil Steril* **41**; 558-63.
17. Tsin DA, Mahmood D (1993). Laparoscopic and hysteroscopic approach for tubal anastomosis. *J Laparoendoc Surg* **3**; 63-6.
18. Sedbon E, Delajolinieres JB, Boudouris O, Madelenat P (1989). Tubal desterilization through exclusive laparoscopy. *Hum Reprod* **4**: 158-9.
19. Istre O, Olsboe F, Trolle B (1993). Laparoscopic tubal anastomosis: reversal of sterilization. *Acta Obstet Gynecol Scand* **72**; 680-1.
20. Nowroozi K, Chase JS, Check JH, Wu CH (1987). The importance of laparoscopic coagulation of mild endometriosis in infertile women. *Int J Fertil* **57**: 442-4.
21. Anonymous (1995). Prospective, randomized double-blind, controlled trial of laser laparoscopy against placebo in stages I-III endometriosis: one year follow-up data.
22. Cook AS, Rock JA (1991). The role of laparoscopy in treatment of endometriosis. *Fertil Steril* **55**; 663-80.
23. Sutton CJG (1993). Lasers in infertility. *Hum Reprod* **8**: 133-46.
24. Gjönnaess H (1984). Polycystic ovarian syndrome treated by ovarian electrocautery through the laparoscope. *Fertil Steril* **41**: 20-5.
25. Dahlgren E (1992). Women with polycystic ovary syndrome wedge resected in 1956 to 1965: a long-term focusing on natural history and circulating hormones. *Fertil Steril* **57**: 505-30.
26. Gaucherand P, Awada A, Rudigoz RC, Dargent D (1994). Obstetrical prognosis of the septate uterus: a plea for treatment of the septum. *Eur J Obstet Gynecol Reprod Biol* **54**: 109-12.
27. Cararach M, Penella J, Ubeda A, Labistida R (1994). Hysteroscopic incision of the septate uterus: scissors versus resectoscope. *Hum Reprod* **9**: 87-9.
28. Elchalal U, Schenker JG (1994). Hysteroscopic resection of uterus septus versus abdominal metroplasty. *J Am Coll Surg* **178**: 637-44.
29. Choe JK, Baggish MS (1992). Hysteroscopic treatment of septate uterus with Neodymium-YAG laser. *Fertil Steril* **57**: 81-4.
30. Rosenfeld DL (1986). Abdominal myomectomy for otherwise unexplained infertility. *Fertil Steril* **46**; 328-30.
31. Gehlbach DL, Sousa RC, Carpenter SE, Rock JA (1993). Abdominal myomectomy in the treatment of infertility. *Int J Gynaecol Obstet* **40**: 45-50.
32. Vollenhoven BJ, Lawrence AS, Healy DL (1990). Uterine fibriods: a clinical review. *Br J Obstet Gynecol* **97**: 285-98.
33. Sutton CJ, Diamond MP (1993). Endoscopic Surgery for Gynaecologists. W.B. Saunders, London.
34. Smith DC, Uhlir JK (1990). Myomectomy as a reproductive procedure. *Am J Obstet Gynecol* **162**: 1476-79.
35. Loffer FD (1990). Removal of large symptomatic intrauterine growths by the hysteroscopic resectoscope. *Obstet Gynecol* **76**: 836-40.
36. Sutton CJ, Whitelaw N (1993) In: Sutton CJ, Diamond MP (eds) Endoscopic Surgery for Gynaecologists. W.B. Saunders, London, pp.159-68.
37. Lichten EM, Bombard J (1987). Surgical treatment of primary dysmenorrhea with laparoscopic uterine nerve ablation. *J Reprod Med* **32**; 37- 41.

Chapter 13
Hysterectomy Techniques
J.H. Phipps

Introduction

Advantages and disadvantages of laparoscopic hysterectomy

Training and patient selection

Terminology

Techniques

Staples and stents
Supracervical laparoscopic hysterectomy
Garry's laparoscopically assisted Doderlein hysterectomy
Classic Semm abdominal hysterectomy

Conclusion

Summary

References

Introduction

This chapter reviews some of the major reservations about the laparoscopic approach to hysterectomy and provides practical descriptions of four of the common surgical approaches.

Advantages and disadvantages of laparoscopic hysterectomy

The possibility of facilitating vaginal hysterectomy by laparoscopic resection of the adnexa and parametrial structures has generated considerable interest over the last few years[1–5]. However, it has yet to be decided by the gynaecological community as a body whether this application of laparoscopic techniques is a viable and useful procedure rather than an expensive gimmick[6], although the tide of opinion seems to be almost universally shifting more towards acceptance rather than rejection. Since the early demonstration of the feasibility of laparoscopically assisted vaginal hysterectomy (LAVH), the laparoscopic approach has gained increasingly wide acceptance throughout Europe and North America[7,8].

Reservations about laparoscopic hysterectomy

- Expense
- Usefulness
- Time required
- High complication rate

The fact that over 80% of hysterectomies in the UK are performed via a laparotomy incision[9] is testament to the inaccuracy of the oft-claimed cry 'I can do it all vaginally' – a major concern of those unconvinced of the merits of laparoscopic hysterectomy.

Key point

Over 80% of hysterectomies performed in the UK involve a laparotomy.

The majority of gynaecologists, when faced with a patient requiring hysterectomy where the uterus is over 12 weeks gestational size, there is a combination of poor vaginal access (due to a narrow pubic arch) and no uterine descent, there is also an indication for oophorectomy, there are known or suspected adhesions in the pelvis (Figure 13.1), or there exist a combination of these factors, usually select open hysterectomy with or without salpingo-oophorectomy. It is rare for gynaecologists to elect to operate vaginally in the UK and the USA where there is a need to remove ovaries, although some workers have demonstrated that this is possible with great facility[10].

The second major concern about these new procedures is the length of the operation. One often hears of a laparoscopic total hysterectomy and bilateral salpingo-oophorectomy requiring two or more hours to complete. This need not be the case. With practice, the operation can usually be completed in around 45 min or less in uncomplicated cases, provided the precepts of Doyen are adhered to. The minimum number of instruments consistent with safe and efficient surgery should be employed. There is never any need, for example, to coagulate with one method (e.g. Nd-YAG laser) and cut with another (e.g. carbon dioxide laser or harmonic scalpel). Straightforward application of endoscopic staples, sutures or bipolar diathermy coagulation and combined cutting and coagulating diathermy-armed instruments are all that is required for the techniques described in this chapter. Bipolar diathermy and sutures are cheaper, but may prolong operation time and, in the case of 'diathermy-only' operations, the possibility of lateral thermal conduction and excessive tissue necrosis must be guarded against.

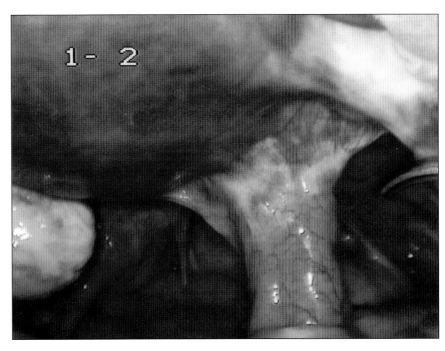

Figure 13.1 *Dense adhesion of small bowel to the right posterior aspect of the uterus, due to operative uterine perforation 2 years before, seen during laparoscopic hysterectomy. Attempted unassisted vaginal hysterectomy may have led to bowel injury.*

Also of relevance to operation time is the question of the ureters. There is little doubt that one of the most common complications of laparoscopic hysterectomy is ureteric injury[11]. Meticulous identification of the ureters by dissection and isolation is very time consuming. Where ureteric anatomy is a cause for concern, the placing of transilluminating ureteric stents for identification is safe, effective and requires less than 2 min (with practice) to perform. We routinely stent the ureters in all hysterectomies, and this is now becoming more widely practised. Hysterectomy techniques in which the cervix is conserved in one way or another[12] constitute less of a risk to the ureter, because the dissection does not proceed lower than the cervicoisthmic junction, at least in theory. The anatomical course of the ureter is notoriously variable, however, and great care must be taken not to damage it when securing haemostasis, particularly with diathermy.

The alternative method making certain of ureteric security is to dissect out the structure, either laparoscopically (as in the original classic technique described by Reich et al.[5]) or (in a laparoscopically assisted Doderlein-type procedure as described by Garry[13]) transvaginally, as it runs underneath the uterine artery.

What follows is to some degree a personal view of the subject. The first technique described here ('staples and stents') has been evolved in our unit over 4 years and some 500 cases. Our rate of significant complication (i.e. where blood transfusion and/or return to theatre is required at some stage) is less than 1% (four of 445 cases) when patients are included only if they underwent our definitive technique. Four techniques are described here, and comprise the four main basic approaches currently in use in this country. I have not included Reich's original technique because the operations described here are the products of evolution from the original. There can be little doubt, however, that in large part we owe the original concept of avoiding laparotomy for the purpose of hysterectomy to Reich[5], one of the great masters of laparoscopic hysterectomy.

Training and patient selection

It is of paramount importance that every step possible should be taken to minimize complications. There can be little doubt that the very best way to achieve this is by properly conducted and adequate training of

---

Key points for safe practice

- Training
- Experience
- Patient selection

---

gynaecologists (as in other surgical specialities) in the skills necessary for safe practice in endoscopy. This issue is currently the focus of attention of both the Royal College of Obstetricians and Gynaecologists and the Department of Health (see Chapters 2 and 3).

The other, and equally vital, prerequisite to successful endoscopic surgery is patient selection. Patients must obviously be offered operations that are appropriate both to the disease and to the ability of the surgeon's stage of training. Attempting a laparoscopic hysterectomy in the presence of severe endometriosis, or where the uterus is of over 12 weeks gestational size, before the surgeon is fully experienced is nothing short of madness, and can only end in disaster. Laparoscopic hysterectomy (in the author's opinion) is probably not appropriate for the treatment of malignant disease with the exception of stage I endometrial carcinoma[14] (J.M. Monaghan, G. Robertson, A.B. Lopez, personal communication), unless (possibly) in the hands of a super-specialist. However, many leading authorities do not agree on this point, and laparoscopic Wertheim's hysterectomy is not an uncommon operation in several centres in Europe.

This chapter is not about training or patient selection, and it is assumed that the endoscopic surgeons and their peers are satisfied that they are adequately trained and experienced.

The indications for a laparoscopic approach to hysterectomy (listed below) include a valid indication for removing the uterus and/or ovaries, circumstances such that simple vaginal hysterectomy is likely to prove difficult, dangerous or impossible, and uterine size not more than 12 weeks gestational size (until considerable experience has been gained).

Contraindications are generally relative to the practice and experience of the surgeon, but include malignancy other than stage I endometrial carcinoma (but see above), uterine size greater than (about) 18 weeks gestational size (and this limit only in the hands of the expert endoscopic surgeon), and the presence of very severe adhesive disease involving the bowel or urinary tract (unless the surgeon is highly expert and is absolutely satisfied at the end of the operation that the bowel, in particular, is intact). It may be noted that, where the large bowel is involved in adhesions below the level of the proximal sigmoid colon, it may be gently transilluminated with any illuminated scope, guided by the exploring finger transrectally, if integrity is in question. This manoeuvre is only for the very experienced, however, as the bowel may easily be perforated if explored inexpertly in this manner.

Terminology

Different, and loosely interchangeable, terms abound in the fields of laparoscopy and hysterectomy, and some authors have chosen to call

---

Indications for laparoscopic hysterectomy

- Valid indication for hysterectomy
- Straightforward vaginal hysterectomy is not possible
- Uterus of less than 18 weeks gestational size

Contraindications to laparoscopic hysterectomy

- Malignant disease
- Severe adhesions
- Uterus of greater than 18 weeks gestational size

---

all of this group of operations 'laparoscopic-vaginal hysterectomy'. However, most authorities would now accept that the term 'laparoscopically assisted vaginal hysterectomy' should be confined to operations in which the laparoscopic dissection stops short of the uterine artery. This would include operations in which the laparoscope is merely used to make sure that no adhesive disease exists prior to straightforward vaginal hysterectomy, and those in which the infundibulopelvic ligaments are dissected and the rest of the operation is completed vaginally. Garry's 'laparoscopic Doderlein's hysterectomy'[13] is a good example of this.

The disadvantage of such operations is that when the uterus is large (16 weeks gestational size or over) and/or there is poor vaginal access, the uterine artery may sometimes be awkward or impossible to secure vaginally. The advantage of the LAVH approach is reduction in operating time for those who operate transvaginally faster than laparoscopically.

Operations that include dissection of the uterine artery and beyond via the laparoscope are referred to as 'laparoscopic hysterectomy'. In the author's experience, it is rarely necessary to dissect laparoscopically beyond the parametrium just inferior to the uterine arteries, as a simple vaginal circumcision of the cervix usually suffices to lift out the uterus with or without the ovaries. In certain cases (typically older patients, virgo intacta or nulliparous with severe atrophic vaginitis), however, it is preferable to complete the whole of the dissection laparoscopically, including the uterosacral ligaments and vaginal skin. The uterus may then be extracted vaginally, with or without morcellation transvaginally, or laparoscopically (which, despite the best efforts of engineers, continues to be a tedious procedure). A morcellator is shown in Figure 13.2.

Techniques

Staples and stents

The standard technique (after Phipps) that we use is as follows[15-17]. A 10 mm trocar and cannula (metal) is inserted beneath the umbilicus to allow passage of the 10 mm laparoscope. Pre-insufflation using a Veress needle is still favoured by some surgeons, but direct entry into the abdomen with the 10 mm trocar and cannula is equally safe and probably safer, although this remains a point of contention. The abdomen is not filled with gas at this point, but the laparoscope is inserted and intraperitoneal fat or bowel (which are recognizable, with practice, without difficulty) must be seen at the end of the laparoscope, to make certain that the cannula is in the correct location, before insufflation. Filling the layers of the abdominal wall, or a hollow viscus or blood vessel, with carbon dioxide then becomes virtually impossible.

The abdomen is insufflated using a high-flow insufflator unit. Two 12 mm trocar and cannulae are passed into the abdominal cavity under direct vision, lateral to the rectus sheaths (Figure 13.3). The inferior epigastric vessels are avoided by direct laparoscopic inspection of the interior abdominal wall. The large vessels of the abdominal wall are almost always visible, and lie just lateral to the peritoneal folds of the obliterated umbilical vessels (Figure 13.4). It is vital that

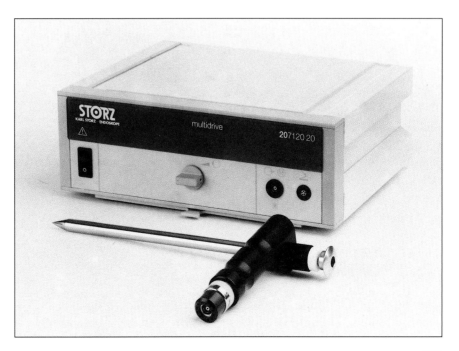

Figure 13.2 *A morcellator.*

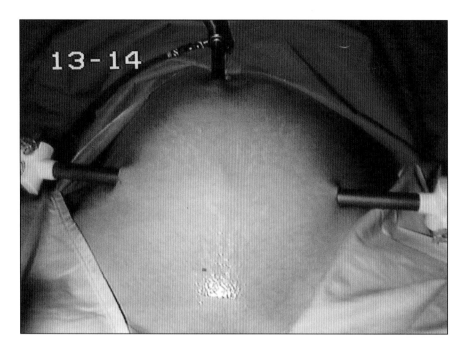

Figure 13.3 *Laparoscopic port cannulae* in situ. *Note the metal cannula for the laparoscope and the absence of plastic skin grips from the lower (metal) cannulae. Bowel burns due to capacitative coupling or accidental shorting of diathermy to the laparoscope cannot occur.*

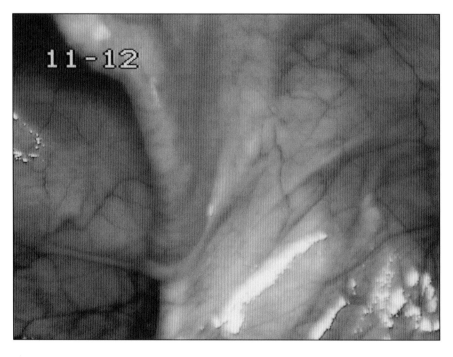

Figure 13.4 *The peritoneal folds of the obliterated right umbilical vessels, and (to the side), the inferior epigastric vessels.*

transillumination of the abdominal wall is not relied on to avoid damage to the inferior epigastric vessels. An assistant cannulates the cervix using either a Hegar dilator and vulsellum (cheaper) or one of the commercially available purpose-built instruments.

If the uterus is very enlarged with fibroids, a fourth 5 mm entry point in the midline, about 4 cm below the laparoscope, may be made for the introduction of a laparoscopic myomectomy screw (Figure 13.5).

The uterus is then displaced by the assistant to the contralateral side to the initial operative site to allow maximum access. The ovarian

Figure 13.5 *The laparoscopic myomectomy screw (4 mm diameter instrument) used to gain access to the parametrium in the presence of large fibroids.*

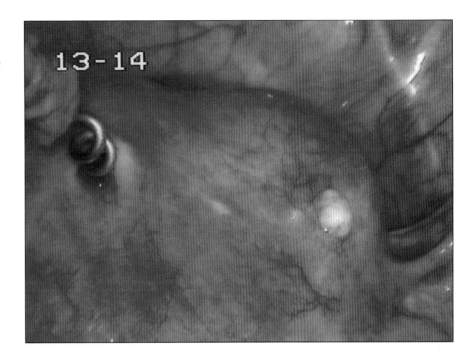

ligament is grasped using laparoscopic forceps via the lower cannula on the opposite side to the initial operating site, and the ovary and tube placed on stretch to expose the infundibulopelvic ligament. The staple gun (EndoGIA 30, Auto Suture, Ascot, UK) is fitted with the 1.0 mm closure height staple cartridge (white-coded), and the infundibulopelvic ligament clamped up to, and preferably over, the round ligament. If the gun jaws fail to close with only moderate pressure on the closure handle, the tissue trapped is excessive and the gun must be removed from the abdomen and fitted with a blue-coded cartridge (1.5 mm closure height). In my opinion, this is the only safe and totally reliable method of achieving perfect haemostasis on every firing of the staple gun. The use of the tissue thickness gauge (EndoGauge, Auto Suture) or similar devices should not be recommended. The accuracy of the device is very poor indeed, and may explain why some surgeons find staples to be an inefficient and unreliable method of securing blood vessels.

At this stage, it is vital to examine the clamped tissues thoroughly (Figure 13.6). The distal tip of the staple gun must be in the 'clear' area of the broad ligament to avoid partial transection of vessels and failure of haemostasis. Care must be taken to avoid the bladder edge and 'tenting' of the pelvic sidewall peritoneum to exclude the possibility of damage to the bladder or ureter. In our experience, there is rarely need to dissect the round and infundibulopelvic ligaments separately. If, however, the round ligament is excluded from this first stapling, it may be included in the diathermy/scissors dissection for the bladder. Ensuring that the tip of the staple gun does not extend below the 'bare' area of the broad ligament, and that the jaws of the instrument are closed immediately lateral to the ovary (i.e. as far from the pelvic

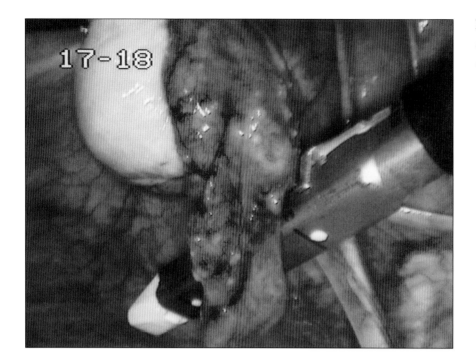

Figure 13.6 *EndoGIA staple gun applied to the infundibulopelvic ligament.*

sidewall as possible), ensures that the ureter is clear of the operative site. We routinely insert transilluminating ureteric stents (Uriglow, Rocket, London, UK; Figure 13.7) cystoscopically at the beginning of the operation, which means that the ureter is easily identified as a row of glowing points[18]. A 25–30° operating cystoscope with an operating channel at least 2 mm in diameter, without manipulation bridge, should be used. The stents should be handled with care to avoid kinking and damage to the fibre optic strands, which may cause spillage of light from cracks and thus a loss in light intensity inside the ureter. It is important that the stents are lubricated with sterile water-soluble jelly to facilitate easy insertion and minimize trauma to the ureters. The stents are

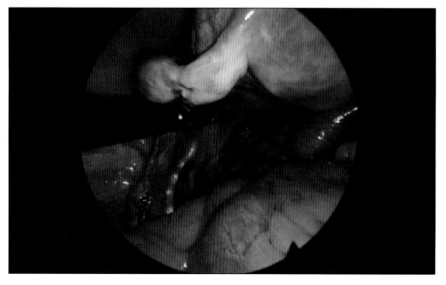

Figure 13.7 *Laparoscopic view of a lighted section of the ureters during hysterectomy.*

graduated with blue lines at 10 mm intervals so that depth of insertion may be judged. There is also a red marker which should lie at or close to the urethral meatus allowing accurate placement. Final adjustment of the stent position may be accomplished under laparoscopic control. Under no circumstances should the stent be advanced too far, as this raises the possibility of traumatizing the renal calyces. Occasionally, light haematuria may be noted for a few hours after operation, but this may be avoided by gentle insertion. The light points running parallel to the uterosacral ligaments must be fully mobile when the staple gun is fully closed over the uterine artery. It is this mobility of the lights that guarantees ureteric freedom from injury. As critics are keen to point out, the ureter is not visible in the ureteric canal. It is not meant to be so: movement of the visible portion is the key to ureteric guarding.

When the surgeon is satisfied that the gun is placed correctly, it may be fired. The bladder is then dissected free and displaced inferiorly and laterally, and the gun placed over the uterine artery, staying clear of the bladder and ureter (Figure 13.8).

When stapling the uterine artery pedicle, it is essential that the jaws remain in the clamped position for a minimum of 1 min prior to firing to allow the entrapped tissues to be compressed and tissue fluid expressed. This ensures good staple fixation and therefore haemostasis. Adequate tissue compression may be judged when the tissues either side of the jaws of the staple gun appear whitish and devascularized. Once again, the staple gun jaws should not be excessively loaded with tissue. Premature firing of the gun may lead to loss of haemostasis. The process is repeated on the opposite side.

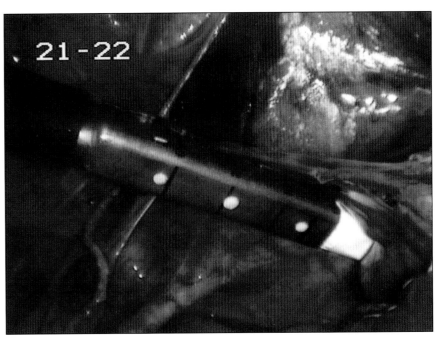

Figure 13.8 *EndoGIA staple gun applied to the uterine artery.*

Key point

It is essential that the jaws of the EndoGIA staple gun remain in the clamped position for a minimum of 1 min prior to firing to allow the entrapped tissues to be compressed and tissue fluid expressed. This ensures good staple fixation and therefore haemostasis.

Using a non-self-locking forceps and scissors, the bladder is then freed from the anterior wall of the uterus, uniting the inferior ends of the incisions achieved with the staple gun. Bladder dissection then proceeds until the vaginal wall is reached. This may be verified by the assistant placing a finger in the anterior fornix; the vagina, stripped free from bladder, is easily identified by the surgeon. It is important at this stage not to incise the vaginal wall because this will cause loss of pneumoperitoneum.

At this stage, the laparoscopic dissection is complete. Although it is possible to divide the uterosacral ligaments and divide the vagina from the cervix circumferentially via the laparoscope, this is more easily achieved vaginally. Moreover, completing the operation vaginally obviates the need to use further endoscopic staples or suturing techniques, reducing operative time and cost.

The laparoscopic ports should be left *in situ* to allow inspection of the uterine bed at the end of the procedure to ensure haemostasis and perform peritoneal toilet.

The vaginal dissection may then be started. It is essential that the surgeon's assistants are aware of the special need for avoiding excessive traction when completing this phase of the operation. Without the support of the round and infundibulopelvic ligaments, the smaller branches of the uterine artery are easily sheared off from the lateral aspect of the body of the uterus, leading to bleeding that may be very difficult indeed to control. This is by far the most common cause of bleeding. The ureteric stents should remain in place until vaginal dissection is finished because, if haemostasis is not secure by the time the uterus is completely removed and extra sutures are needed to control bleeding from the uterine artery pedicles, it is possible to damage or obstruct the ureter at this stage.

The cervix is grasped using two pairs of vulsellum forceps, and the dissection proceeds much as for vaginal hysterectomy, although certain aspects require emphasis. The pouch of Douglas is opened using a knife to incise the posterior fornix vaginal skin and peritoneum. Circumcision of the cervix is then completed circumferentially, and the uterovesical pouch opened to unite with the laparoscopic bladder dissection. Once entry is gained to the peritoneal cavity, both anteriorly and posteriorly, the bladder (and therefore the ureters) should be displaced laterally and superiorly to ensure that the urinary tract is clear of the operative field. With uretic stents *in situ* the ureters may be easily palpated and avoided.

The exploring finger is then placed through the peritoneum anteriorly, into the uterovesical pouch, and curled around the remaining tissue (mostly comprising the transverse cervical ligaments) and the finger tip exited through the ipsilateral incision in the pouch of Douglas. A long, curved-on-the-edge non-toothed clamp (ideally a 30 cm Zeppelin clamp) is then placed over the tissue in a single manoeuvre. Occasionally, this volume of tissue will prove excessive for a single clamp, and may have to be dealt with in two stages. The uterus is then delivered vaginally, taking care to rotate it through 90° to avoid snagging the lateral pelvic sidewall staples (see below). If the uterus is grossly enlarged, it may be bisected and morcellated in the usual way.

The uterine bed should then be thoroughly inspected vaginally for bleeding. Sometimes, it is possible to visualize the whole of the dissection, including the staples in the infundibulopelvic ligament, but more often the latter requires laparoscopic inspection. If extra sutures are required to secure a leaking pedicle, special care must be taken laterally to avoid the ureters.

If the uterus is enlarged by fibroids to an extent that extracting the uterus through the pelvic outlet is likely to prove difficult, the possibility of snagging the staples on the infundibulopelvic and uterine artery pedicles must be borne in mind. The sides of the isolated uterus are also studded with staples, which may catch and even avulse those securing the pedicles, leading to potentially severe bleeding. This may be avoided by rotating the isolated uterus through 90° before extraction. The two lines of staples on the uterus and pelvic sidewall are thereby separated, and snagging avoided.

It is my experience that there is no need to close the peritoneum separately, although it should be included in the vaginal skin stitch posteriorly to prevent bleeding from the usually very vascular space between the layers of the vaginal skin and peritoneum. I favour the use of a transvaginal tube drain, left through the vault for 24 h. Although there is usually no need to use a vaginal pack for haemostasis, packing of the vagina makes subsequent laparoscopic inspection of the uterine bed easier, as it 'tents' the vault, exposes the dissection line and seals the vagina against loss of gas for the final inspection. Bladder catheterization for 24 h enables the patient to rest without getting out of bed, but this must be balanced against the increased risk of urinary tract infection.

The abdomen is re-insufflated, and the uterine bed checked for bleeding. Insufflation pressure should be kept to a minimum consistent with good visualization because higher pressures may conceal venous leakage. Any leaking vessel may be dealt with using bipolar diathermy, although the possible proximity of the ureters must always be kept in mind. It is very important to avoid applying unipolar diathermy to tissue bearing staples. If current is applied directly to the staple line, the tissue immediately surrounding each staple will necrose, resulting in potential loss of haemostasis. A final check may be made in the absence of a pneumoperitoneum using the C abdominal wall retractor[19] (Figure 13.9). Finally, the ports are closed with a J peritoneal closure needle[20] (Figure 13.10).

This technique has a long and extensive track record for safety and speed in the operating theatre (see above). It is interesting that, of students on the George Eliot Minimal Access Gynaecological Training Centre laparoscopic hysterectomy course who go on to complete their training and take up laparoscopic hysterectomy in their own units, almost all expressed a preference for this technique compared with the alternatives. The disadvantage is cost: disposables per case run at about £490 including stents. However, a single ureteric injury in 1000 cases would outweigh the cost of stenting all 1000 cases, in terms of re-operation and subsequent medicolegal problems. We believe that the safety and consistent results of this procedure justify the expense.

Supracervical laparoscopic hysterectomy

Sutton's technique is basically a modification of Semm's CASH operation. The main difference is that staples are used instead of endoscopic sutures. At the beginning of the operation, the cervicouterine canal is cannulated, and a coaxial boring bar-type instrument is used to core out the cervix to just above the level of the isthmus. This removes the transformation zone, and is an answer to the problem of possible future development of malignancy in the

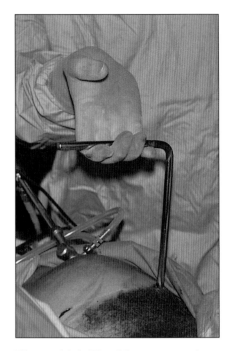

Figure 13.9 *The C-bar retractor in use.*

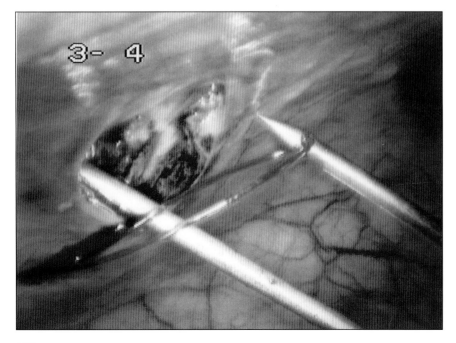

Figure 13.10 *Closure of lateral port wounds with J peritoneal closure needle[21].*

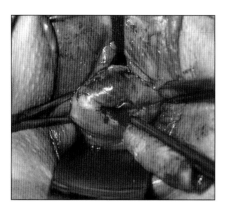

Figure 13.11 *A core of tissue including the transformation zone is removed during a supracervical laparoscopic hysterectomy.*

cervical stump. Once this is achieved, the infundibulopelvic and broad ligaments are dealt with laparoscopically, to a level just above the uterine artery. The uterus is then divided, isthmus from cervix, with a laser, harmonic scalpel or diathermy, and the uterine body removed by morcellation via one of the abdominal ports. Figure 13.11 shows a core of tissue being removed from the cervix.

The vagina is not opened, and this carries the great advantage of operative sterility. Other advantages are that the ureters are safe, because they are not approached by the staple gun as they lie under the uterine arteries, and the cervix is conserved.

The philosophy underlying this technique is that of cervical conservation. The claimed advantages of not removing the cervix in terms of sexual function (particularly female orgasm) have never been proved (although they are currently under investigation by Sutton's team). If one contends that removal of the cervix condemns the patient to anorgasmia or, at best, dysorgasmia, presumably one must also cite uterosacral nerve ablation (often performed in relatively young women) and vaginal hysterectomy as being culprits in terms of sexual maiming. The issue remains contentious.

Operative time for this procedure is reported at being around an hour and a half, but this must depend on the size of the uterus and how much morcellation has to be performed. Despite ingenious engineering developments in motorizing morcellation devices, it remains to some degree time consuming. Nevertheless, this technique has been used with great success and avoids the need to stent the ureters (although beware the sometimes deviant path of the ureter which can bring it into the operative field of the infundibulopelvic ligament). In terms of cost, the technique is in the mid-range, because some staples are usually employed (although one firing per side instead of the two described above).

Garry's laparoscopically assisted Doderlein's hysterectomy technique (Figures 13.12 (a) to (j)).

This technique (after Garry) relies firstly on a laparoscopic approach to deal with any adhesions and to divide the infundibulopelvic and broad ligaments as far as the uterine artery, but no further. Once the upper pedicles are dealt with, by bipolar diathermy (or extracorporeally knotted sutures), the bulk of the operation is performed vaginally. An incision is made on the anterior vaginal wall extending from the 9 o'clock to the 3 o'clock position. The bladder is then dissected free from the anterior surface of the uterus, and pushed up and laterally, taking the ureters with it. A Wertheim's retractor is then inserted between the bladder and uterus. The anterior surface of the uterus is grasped using a vulsellum forceps, as cephalad as possible, and traction is applied. Simultaneously, a vulsellum forceps on the posterior lip of the cervix is pushed upward to create a rocking movement of the uterus, to deliver the fundus of the uterus into the vagina through the uterovesical pouch. The uterine arteries are then exposed and lie inferior to the ureters, which may also be identified. This is the alternative to either avoiding the ureters completely (or at least attempting to do so) as in supracervical hysterectomy, or stenting them.

Very good results have been reported for this technique: Saye et al.[21] claim a mean operating time of about an hour, with most patients leaving hospital within 23 h.

Figure 13.12 *Garry's laparoscopically assisted Doderlein's hysterectomy*

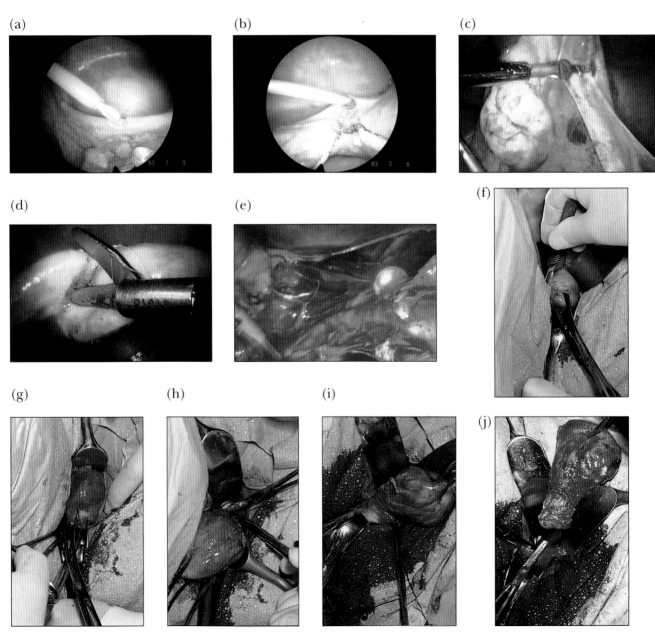

Garry is able to deal with moderately large uteri using this technique, which has the great advantage of cheapness. He uses no disposable instruments, and has a good safety record. Thinking of the uterine inversion manoeuvre, however, one wonders what size of uterus with what degree (or lack) of prolapse could be dealt with in this manner without risking shearing off the uterine arteries from the pelvic sidewall, a notoriously difficult problem to deal with if it occurs. Manipulating a large non-prolapsed uterus vaginally is not at all a difficult or bloody event if the uterine arteries have been dealt with from above.

Classic Semm abdominal hysterectomy

No description of laparoscopic techniques would be complete without including this product of the great master, Professor Kurt Semm. This procedure is the father of Sutton's technique, but Semm specifies the use of sutures rather than staples. The obvious advantage is in terms of cost, but the price one pays for this is reduced speed of operation. The technique for boring out the cervix is exactly the same.

It is worth mentioning that extreme care must be taken not to deviate from the midline, particularly in the coronal plane, because massive haemorrhage, and broad ligament haematoma that is difficult to deal with, will result from boring into the sides of the uterus. The axial course of the boring bar is, however, guided by a midline ream, which deliberately perforates the uterus at the fundus as this minimizes the risk of damage to the large uterine vessels.

Conclusion

It is my contention that these techniques should never be in competition, but should be viewed as complementary. Different surgeons and different patients may warrant the use of one in preference to another, depending on the circumstances. Flexibility in surgical practice is to be applauded. It is rare that a single egocentric view of medicine is the only correct one; truth usually lies in a blend of perspectives. The flexible, and therefore able, surgeon is familiar with aspects of all available techniques, to be better armed to cope with any situation or case that may arise.

There are many variations on the theme of laparoscopic hysterectomy, but limitation of space prevents description of them all. I have not described techniques that require an operating time of several hours, because few surgeons in the UK have the time (or the inclination) to indulge in such procedures. Similarly, I have omitted techniques that seem either potentially dangerous or at least unreliable. It is my contention that, at present, there is little place for laparoscopic surgery in the management of advanced malignancy, although laparoscopic node sampling to decide on future surgical treatment may be the exception to the rule. Struggling to remove large fibroid uteri or vast ovarian cysts simply to prove technical feasibility, likewise, can surely have no sane supporter.

Summary

Although there is a general shift towards laparoscopic hysterectomy as the operation of choice, it is still seen by many clinicians as a controversial procedure; the main concerns being expense, operating time and high complication rates. The author argues that these obstacles can be overcome by a combination of thorough training, experience and a critical approach to patient selection.

The indications and contraindications for laparoscopic hysterectomy are discussed with clear guidance given on surgical technique, stapling procedures and equipment. Pioneering operations such as the laparoscopically assisted Doderlein's hysterectomy and the classic Semm abdominal hysterectomy are described.

Finally, it is suggested that in the best interest of patient safety surgeons should retain a flexible approach to the various operations in their armamentarium and not restrict themselves to one particular procedure.

References

1. Scrimgeour JB, Ng KB, Gaudion MR (1981) Laparoscopy in vaginal hysterectomy. *Lancet* **338**: 1465–6 (letter).
2. Magos AL, Broadbent JA, Amso NN (1991) Laparoscopically assisted vaginal hysterectomy. *Lancet* **338**: 1091–2 (letter).
3. Reich H (1989) New techniques in advanced laparoscopic surgery. *Baillieres Clin Obstet Gynaecol* **3**: 655–81.
4. Reich H, McGlynn F, Wilkie W (1990) Laparoscopic management of stage ovarian cancer. *J Reprod Med* **35**: 601–4.
5. Reich H, DeCaprio J, McGlynn F (1989) Laparoscopic hysterectomy. *J Gynecol Surg* **5**: 213–16.
6. RCOG (1993). The laparoscopic approach to hysterectomy is unnecessary? Royal College of Obstetricians and Gynaecologists Conference on Endoscopic Gynaecological Surgery. RCOG, London.
7. Bruhat MA, Mage G, Chapron JL, Pouly JL, Canis M, Wattiez A (1991) Present day endoscopic surgery in gynecology. *Eur J Obstet Gynecol Reprod Biol* **41**: 4–13.
8. Nezhat F, Nezhat C, Gordon S, Wilkins E (1992) Laparoscopic *versus* abdominal hysterectomy. *J Reprod Med* **37**: 247–50.
9. Sutton C (1992) Operative laparoscopy. *Curr Opin Obstet Gynaecol* **4**: 430–8.
10. Sheth S, Malpani A (1992) Routine prophylactic oophorectomy at the time of vaginal hysterectomy in post-menopausal women. *Arch Gynecol Obstet* **251**: 87–91.

11. Woodland MB (1992) Ureter injury during laparoscopy-assisted vaginal hysterectomy with the endoscopic linear stapler. *Am J Obstet Gynecol* **167**: 756–7.

12. Semm K (1993) Hysterectomy by pelviscopy: an alternative approach without colpotomy (CASH). In: Garry R, Reich H (eds) *Laparoscopic Hysterectomy.* Blackwell Scientific, Oxford, pp. 118–32.

13. Garry R (1994) The evolution of a technique for laparoscopic hysterectomy: laparoscopic-assisted Doderlein's hysterectomy. *Gynaecol Endosc* **3**: 123–8.

14. Phipps JH, Monaghan JM (1993) Laparoscopic hysterectomy and cancer. *Surg Oncol* (Suppl 1): 67–72.

15. Phipps JH (1993) *Laparoscopic Hysterectomy and Oophorectomy: A Practical Manual and Colour Atlas.* Churchill Livingstone, Edinburgh, p. 14.

16. Phipps JH, John M, Nayak S (1993) Laparoscopically-assisted vaginal hysterectomy and bilateral salpingoophorectomy *versus* open abdominal hysterectomy and bilateral salpingoophorectomy. *Br J Obstet Gynaecol* **100**: 668–70.

17. Phipps JH, John M, Saeed M, Hassanien M (1993) Laparoscopic and laparoscopically-assisted vaginal hysterectomy: a series of 144 cases. *Gynaecol Endosc* **2**: 7–12.

18. Phipps JH, Tyrrell NJ (1991) Transilluminating ureteric stents for preventing operative ureteric injury. *Br J Obstet Gynaecol* **99**: 81.

19. Phipps JH (1993) 'C bar' abdominal wall suspension retractor for laparoscopic surgery without positive pressure pneumoperitoneum. *Gynaecol Endosc* **2**: 183–4.

20. Phipps JH, Taranissi M (1994) Laparoscopic peritoneal closure needle for prevention of port herniae and management of abdominal wall vessel injury. *Gynaecol Endosc* **3**: 189–91.

21. Saye WB, Espey GB, Bishop MR, Miller WM, Hertzman P (1993) Laparoscopic Doderlein hysterectomy: a rational alternative to traditional abdominal hysterectomy. *Surg Laparosc Endosc* **3**: 88–94.

Chapter 14
Laparoscopic Colposuspension
A.R.B. Smith

Introduction

The number of procedures described to cure stress incontinence of urine is considerable, reflecting a failure to produce a procedure with low patient morbidity and high long-lasting cure rate. This chapter reviews the development of bladder neck surgery leading up to and including laparoscopic colposuspension. The technique is described including difficulties and how to avoid complications.

Management of stress incontinence

Many surgical procedures designed to cure stress incontinence have been described. Unfortunately, although the number of procedures described is large, the number of controlled studies with objective preoperative and postoperative assessment with long-term follow-up is small. This makes comparison of the relative merits of procedures difficult.

During the past 45 years, there have been two major developments in the management of stress incontinence. Firstly, the increasing use of preoperative urodynamic assessment has led to a reduction in the number of patients with abnormal bladder function having inappropriate bladder neck surgery. Secondly, concern about the high risk of recurrence of stress incontinence following vaginal surgery has led to increased use of the abdominal–retropubic approach, which allows greater bladder neck elevation, gives a higher success rate and reduces the risk of recurrence.

Increasing experience with retropubic bladder neck suspension procedures has led to the recognition that the higher cure rate may be accompanied by an increased risk of postoperative voiding difficulty, detrusor instability and vaginal prolapse. In addition, employment of minimally invasive techniques for colposuspension such as described by Pereyra[1] and Stamey[2] have not produced results as good or as long lasting as with the conventional colposuspension first described by Burch[3] in 1961. To date, there are insufficient data to determine whether laparoscopic colposuspension represents an advance in the surgical management of stress incontinence in terms of cure and postoperative recovery or merely a further procedure in a long list of procedures that have promised but failed to produce a high cure rate with low morbidity.

Open colposuspension

Burch[3] experienced technical difficulty reproducing the colposuspension described by Marshall *et al.*[4] in which the periurethral

> # Key points in surgical treatment of urinary stress incontinence
>
> - Preoperative urodynamic assessment is essential
> - Retropubic bladder neck suspension gives better elevation and long-term cure than vaginal repair
> - The retropubic approach is associated with voiding difficulty, detrusor instability and vaginal prolapse (enterocele)

fascia was sutured to the periosteum of the pubis. Cooper's ligament proved to be an easier fixed point than either the periosteum of the pubis or the arcus tendineus fascia. Burch[3] reported satisfactory results in 93% of 143 patients, only 12 of whom had undergone previous surgery. No cystometric studies were performed. Burch noted at an early stage that postoperative enterocele was common and incorporated obliteration of the cul de sac into the procedure, but still reported postoperative enterocele in 7.6% of cases. Burch employed no. 2 chromic catgut suture for colposuspension and reported failure of bladder neck suspension in only two of 143 cases at follow-up. Currently, most surgeons prefer a stronger more durable suture material and many employ a non-absorbable suture. No trial has established the optimal suture material. A non-absorbable suture material carries a risk of stone formation if placed or migrated into the bladder.

Numerous reports on Burch colposuspension have been published over the past 35 years, but most do not include a large number of patients with objective preoperative and postoperative assessment with long-term follow-up including documentation of complications. In 1993, Kiilholma et al.[5] reported on a 2 year follow-up of 186 women after colposuspension: 95% of women undergoing colposuspension as a primary procedure were cured or markedly improved compared with 82% who had undergone previous bladder neck surgery; 9% of patients experienced voiding difficulty and 12% of patients developed a rectocele or enterocele after operation; 19% of patients described urinary urgency *de novo*, which is the same incidence of detrusor instability found by Cardozo et al.[6] in a study of 92 patients following colposuspension. Thus, the data indicate that open colposuspension provides a good chance of curing stress incontinence, particularly as a primary procedure, but problems with abnormal bladder function, voiding and vaginal prolapse may follow surgery.

In a 5 year follow-up of 127 women undergoing primary bladder neck surgery, Elia and Bergman[7] reported a higher success rate for colposuspension than for vaginal repair or Stamey procedure. Twice as many women were continent 5 years after colposuspension than after vaginal repair or Stamey procedure (82% vs 37% and 43%, respectively). Alcalay et al.[8] investigated a group of 109 women with a mean follow-up of 14 years following colposuspension. They reported a time-dependent fall in cure rate over 10 years, after which a plateau was reached.

In summary, it would appear that open colposuspension produces the highest success rate with the greatest longevity of cure. The less invasive needle colposuspension, although undoubtedly resulting in less surgical trauma to the patient, appears to result in a lower short-term cure rate and a higher risk of recurrence. All studies indicate that primary surgery is more likely to be successful than subsequent surgery, so there is a good argument for opting for open colposuspension as a primary procedure. Balanced against this, however, must be the incidence of postoperative detrusor instability, voiding dysfunction and vaginal prolapse. Unfortunately, there are no good comparative data on the incidence of these problems, but it would seem logical that voiding dysfunction will become increasingly prevalent with increasing bladder neck elevation. It is possible that the paravaginal defect repair is the compromise approach. Shull and Baden[9] reported a cure rate of 97% for stress incontinence in a series of 149 women undergoing predominantly primary bladder neck surgery. Voiding problems were not encountered, presumably because anatomical distortion is not produced, but vaginal vault prolapse after operation was noted in 6% of patients.

Early experience with laparoscopic colposuspension

The view of the retropubic space through the laparoscope, introduced through or outside the peritoneal cavity, can be excellent. The value of gaining access to the retropubic space in this way, with its shorter convalescence, has to be matched against the capital cost of the equipment, the additional technical expertise required by the surgeon and the risks inherent in laparoscopic surgery. Even if a technically excellent result is achieved by the laparoscopic approach, the early return to normal activity commonly seen in these patients may result in more frequent recurrence of symptoms as reported as with needle colposuspension.

The first report on laparoscopic colposuspension by Vancaillie and Schuessler[10] in 1991 included nine patients. Two of the first four patients required laparotomy to complete the procedure, indicating the technical difficulty of the operation. In 1993, Liu[11] reported on a series of 58 patients who all had demonstrable primary stress incontinence and normal bladder function on simple office cystometry. The intraperitoneal approach was adopted. The

---

Laparoscopic colposuspension

- Better view of the retropubic space
- Shorter convalescence
- Need for greater technical expertise
- No long-term follow-up

---

peritoneum was opened through an incision 2.5–3.5 cm above the symphysis pubis on the anterior abdominal wall between the obliterated hypogastric artery folds in the peritoneum. After bladder mobilization, two GORE-TEX sutures (W.L. Gore, Woking, UK), including a full-thickness double bite in the anterior vaginal wall, were fixed to Cooper's ligament on each side. The peritoneal defect was closed and cystoscopy performed. In the 58 cases reported, one sustained a bladder injury during surgery which was repaired laparoscopically and another bled from a suprapubic catheter insertion. The suprapubic catheter was removed in all cases 1 week after surgery and no cases of voiding difficulties were reported. No patient leaked during a standing stress test 3 months after surgery, but three patients had increased incontinence due to intrusor instability, although it is not clear how this was defined. All patients were allowed to drive and return to work 1 week after surgery provided that their job did not require much physical exertion. It is not made clear what tasks the patients were able to perform or did perform following surgery.

Nezhat *et al.*[12] retrospectively reviewed 62 women who underwent laparoscopic bladder neck surgery as a primary procedure. In 16 patients who either had or were thought likely to develop an enterocele, a Moschowitz procedure[13] was employed. The periurethral fascia was elevated to Cooper's ligament or the midline of the symphysis pubis cartilage depending on the surgeon's preference. A single Ethibond suture (Ethicon, Edinburgh, UK) was used in most cases, additional sutures being placed in only five cases. The peritoneal defect was left open in 40 of 62 cases and closed only when it had become enlarged. One intraoperative bladder injury occurred, which was repaired laparoscopically. Of the 62 patients, 58 were able to void on the second or third postoperative day. Five of 62 patients had symptomatic leakage after operation, four of whom had proven detrusor instability. There were no cases of vaginal prolapse in this series.

To overcome the difficulty of laparoscopic suturing, Ou *et al.*[14] developed a technique of laparoscopic colposuspension using Prolene mesh (Ethicon, Edinburgh, UK) fixed to the paraurethral fascia and Cooper's ligaments with titanium staples. The staples are applied through a disposable hernia stapling gun, the cost of which may be regained through reduced operating time. No failure was reported in a series of 40 patients with a mean of 6 months follow-up. No complications of staples in the anterior vaginal wall were reported.

Another form of laparoscopic colposuspension has been described by Harewood[15]. In a series of seven patients, a Stamey-type procedure was performed under laparoscopic vision. The author suggests that the advantage of the laparoscopic approach is that it allows direct examination of the bladder and observation of the bladder neck during tying of the sutures. Despite this advantage, bladder perforation occurred in one case.

Burton[16] performed the only published randomized controlled trial of laparoscopic and open colposuspension. In a series of 60 patients undergoing primary treatment for stress incontinence, full postoperative subjective and objective assessment was performed at 6 and 12 months. The procedure was performed through the peritoneal cavity, and four polyglycolic acid sutures were placed in all cases. One bladder perforation occurred in each group. Subjectively, six of 30 women from the laparoscopic group leaked urine at 12 months compared with two of 30 in the open colposuspension group. Burton operated on 10 women laparoscopically before the study to familiarize himself with the technique. Many surgeons would suggest that more experience is advisable before conducting such a study. Having performed over 120 laparoscopic colposuspensions, I would suggest that the learning curve is longer than for open surgery, primarily because of the difficulty with suturing. This is well illustrated by a 50% reduction in mean operating time noted over the first 50 cases.

Techniques

Access to the retropubic space
All laparoscopic surgeons need to be aware of the vessels of the anterior abdominal wall as illustrated in Figure 14.1.

Transperitoneal
Optimal port positions for the transperitoneal approach are illustrated in Figures 14.1 and 14.2. The advantages and disadvantages of this approach are listed in Table 14.1.

Extraperitoneal
Optimal port positions are illustrated in Figures 14.1 and 14.2. Under normal conditions, the loose areolar connective tissue of the retropubic space can be divided easily with blunt dissection. Balloon devices are available and may prove helpful.

The main difficulty is avoiding bladder injury. Adhesions from previous pelvic surgery can adhere the bladder to the anterior

Figure 14.1 *Vessels of the anterior abdominal wall and optimal port positions.*
1 = superficial epigastric artery
2 = superficial circumflex artery
3 = inferior epigastric artery
4 = deep circumflex artery

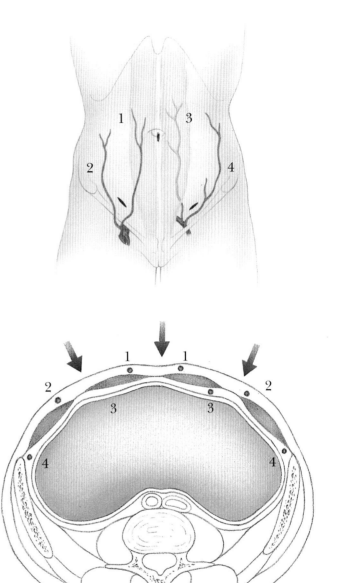

Figure 14.2 *Transverse section of the abdomen showing relationship of port positions and vessels.*

Advantages	Disadvantages
Intraperitoneal procedure	Risk of injury to the inferior epigastric artery
Other procedures possible, including treatment of enterocele	Risk of bowel injury with port insertion
Larger operating field	Risk of bladder injury when opening the peritoneum
	Risk of hernia from portal wounds
	Intraperitoneal adhesions from previous surgery may limit access to the anterior abdominal wall

Table 14.1 *Advantages and disadvantages of the transperitoneal approach*

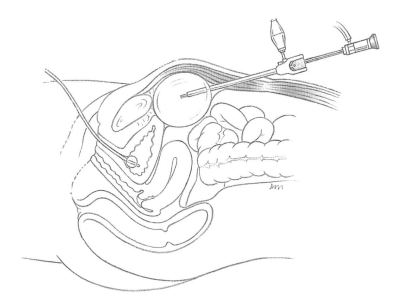

Figure 14.3 *Balloon distension device can be used to dissect the extra peritoneal cavity under direct vision.*

abdominal wall. This can best be overcome by dissection into the retropubic space lateral to the midline at first, because most adhesions from previous surgery occur centrally and are easier to identify when the space has been opened laterally.

Mobilization of periurethral fascia

The surgeon's index finger is placed in the vagina lateral to the bladder neck while the bladder is mobilized medially with the aid of a pledget attached to graspers (Figure 14.4). It is advisable to tie a long suture to the pledget to avoid losing it. Disposable pledgets fixed to a holder are available.

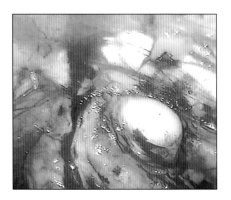

Fixation of periurethral fascia to Cooper's ligament

Using a straight needle attached to a suture of choice, two bites of the periurethral fascia and a single bite of Cooper's ligament are taken and the needle withdrawn. A Roeder knot is tied and pushed down by an assistant, elevating the fascia (Figure 14.5). It is not always possible to attain direct approximation of fascia to ligament, particularly when an anterior vaginal repair has been performed previously. I place two sutures on each side to ensure a strong fixation. The main difference from open colposuspension is that a narrower area of fascia is elevated by the laparoscopic route, although the difference is not detectable on vaginal examination.

If a paravaginal repair is performed, less bladder mobilization is required but a curved needle is necessary to secure fixation to the fascia on the pelvic sidewall.

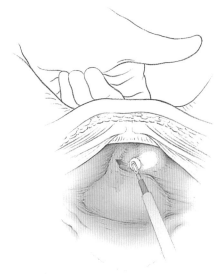

Figure 14.4 *The bladder is mobilized medially with the aid of a pledget attached to grasping forceps.*

Figure 14.5 *A suture is passed through the periurethral fascia and Cooper's ligaments and secured using an extracorporeal Roeder knot.*
(a) Suturing of Cooper's ligament to the anterior vaginal wall.
(b) The suture in place.

Figure 14.5a

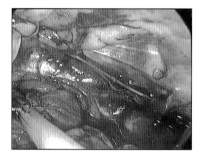

Figure 14.5b

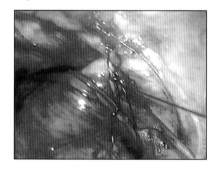

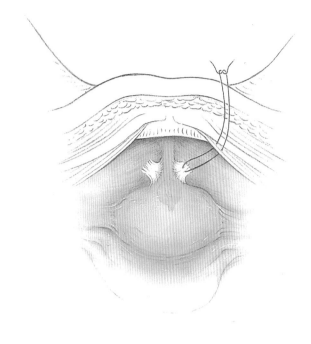

Suprapubic catheterization

I use suprapubic catheterization to ease the management of patients with postoperative voiding difficulties. The bladder is filled via the urethral catheter, which is present throughout surgery on free drainage. The suprapubic catheter is inserted under direct vision into the bladder. A Bonano catheter (Figure 14.6) is suitable, but other types equally serve the purpose.

Figure 14.6 *A Bonano catheter puncturing the bladder under direct vision. (Courtesy of Olympus KeyMed (Medical & Industrial Equipment) Ltd, Southend-on-Sea, UK)*

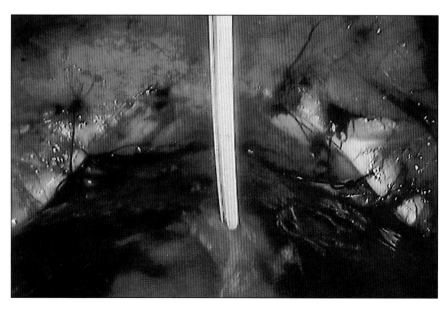

Peritoneal closure

The anterior abdominal peritoneum may be closed, but this is not necessary if the peritoneal incision is large. A narrow gap in the peritoneum could lead to bowel entrapment. In three out of four cases in which I reoperated some months after laparoscopic colposuspension, the peritoneum had healed normally. In the other case, the retropubic space remained open, but had become peritonealized.

Wound closure

There is a significant risk of hernia formation in portal wounds of more than 5 mm diameter. A full-thickness closure is therefore required in lateral wounds of more than 5 mm. Disposable and reusable devices are available for this, as described in earlier chapters.

Postoperative care

Analgesic requirements are variable, but generally much less than for open colposuspension. I clamp the suprapubic catheter 36 h after surgery and remove the suprapubic catheter when the residual urine is less than 150 ml. In my experience, 60% of catheters can be removed by the fourth day, but voiding problems after this are not uncommon. On rare occasions, long-term intermittent self-catheterization is required.

Summary

Early experience with laparoscopically assisted colposuspension has shown that it is possible for perform this procedure safely leading to an early return to normal activities. Although it is possible to achieve a level of reduction of symptoms equivalent to that of open surgery, a decision on the usefulness of this procedure awaits the outcome of 5–10 year follow-up studies. Pre-operative assessment with urodynamic studies is mandatory. It is possible to obtain an excellent view of the retropubic space and the colposuspension procedure can be performed using an intra– or an extra–peritoneal approach. Laparoscopic suturing requires additional skills, but encouraging results have been reported with the use of prolene mesh fixed with titanium staples. Complications are similar in type and frequency to those encountered in open surgery. Post—operative bladder care is similar to that required following open surgery.

References

1. Pereyra AJ (1959) A simplified surgical procedure for the correction of stress urinary incontinence in women. W*estern Journal of Surgery, Obstetrics and Gynaecology* **67**: 223–6.

2. Stamey TA (1973) Endoscopic suspension of the vesical neck for urinary incontinence. *Surg Gynecol and Obstet* **136**: 547–54.

3. Burch JC (1961) Urethrovaginal fixation to Cooper's ligament for correction of stress incontinence, cystocele and prolapse. *Am J Obstet Gynecol* **81**: 281–90.

4. Marshall VF, Marchetti AA, Krantz KE (1949) The correction of stress incontinence by simple vesicourethral suspension. *Surg Gynecol Obstet* **88**: 509–18.

5. Kiilholma P, Makinen J, Chancellor MB, Pitkanen Y, Hirvonen T (1993) Modified Burch colposuspension for stress urinary incontinence in females. *Surg Gynecol Obstet* **176**: 111–15.

6. Cardozo LD, Stanton SI, Williams JE (1979) Detrusor instability following surgery for genuine stress incontinence. *Br J Urol* **51**: 204–7.

7. Elia G, Bergman A (1994) Prospective randomised comparison of three surgical procedures for stress urinary incontinence: five year follow up. *Neurology and Urodynamics* **13**: 498–500.

8. Alcalay M, Monga A, Stanton SL (1994) Burch colposuspension: how long does it cure stress incontinence? *Neurology and Urodynamics* **13**: 495–6.

9. Shull BL, Baden WF (1989) A six year experience with paravaginal defect repair. *Am J Obstet Gynecol* **160**: 1432–40.

10. Vancaillie TG, Schuessler W (1991) Laparoscopic bladder neck suspension. *J Laparoendosc Surg* **1**: 169–73.

11. Liu CY (1993) Laparoscopic retropubic colposuspension (Burch procedure): A review of 58 cases. *J Reprod Med* **38**: 526–30.

12. Nezhat CH, Nezhat F, Nezhat CR, Rottenburg H (1994) Laparoscopic retropubic cystourethropexy. *J Am Assoc Gynecol Laparosc* **1**: 339–49.

13. Moschowitz AV (1912) The pathogenesis, anatomy and cure of prolapse of the rectum. *Surg Gynecol Obstet* **15**: 7.

14. Ou CS, Presthus J, Beadle E (1993) Laparoscopic bladder neck suspension using hernia mesh and surgical staples. *J Laparoendosc Surg* **3**: 563–6.

15. Harewood LM (1993) Laparoscopic needle colposuspension for genuine stress incontinence. *J Endourol* **7**: 319–22.

16. Burton G (1994) A randomised comparison of laparoscopic and open colposuspension. *Neurology and Urodynamics* **13**: 497–8.

Chapter 15

Endometrial Resection and Ablation Using Electrocautery

C.J.G. Sutton

Introduction

This chapter describes in some detail the indications, patient selection and operative technique of endometrial resection. The equipment used is briefly reviewed and in conclusion the surgeon is warned against underestimating the difficulty of the procedure or the potentially fatal complications resulting from inadequate training.

Background

Many people have commented on the extraordinary length of time general surgeons took to adopt the laparoscope, either for diagnosis or for operative surgery, but a similar criticism could equally apply to gynaecologists, many of whom have been working in adjacent operating theatres to their urological colleagues and have watched the operation of transurethral resection of the prostate with a detached fascination, but without the foresight or perspicacity to translate the modus operandi to endoscopic removal of the endometrium. The credit for this must go to Milton Goldrath from Detroit, Michigan, who introduced laser ablation of the endometrium with the Nd-YAG laser[1]. The first reported use of electrosurgical resection was by Robert Neuwirth[2], from New York, who used it to remove symptomatic submucous fibroids, and the first description of endometrial resection by DeCherney and his colleagues[3], who ablated the endometrium in a small series of patients with intractable bleeding who, for one reason or another, were unsuitable for abdominal or vaginal hysterectomy.

Indications and patient selection

Although it has been estimated[4] that up to 58% of women currently being treated by hysterectomy for menstrual dysfunction may be suitable for endometrial resection or ablation, this requires very careful patient selection. The treatment criteria for endometrial ablation are set out in Table 15.1.

Endometrial resection or ablation is an invasive procedure with a definite complication rate, and some of these complications can be serious or fatal, and should therefore never be embarked on lightly. Women must be absolutely certain that they have completed their family and should preferably have had tubal occlusion because pregnancies can occur after this procedure but are often associated with complications, some of which may be serious or even life threatening.

The women should be complaining of severe menorrhagia, sufficient to seriously affect their life style, and should give a history of

Table 15.1 *Criteria for endometrial ablation*

Severe menorrhagia justifying hysterectomy
Failed medical treatment
Family complete
Uterine cavity length <12 cm (14 weeks gestational size)
Benign histology (smear, pipelle, transvaginal ultrasonography or hysteroscopy)
Careful counselling on:
    Amenorrhoea – occurs in only 30% of cases
    Pregnancy avoidance
    Laparoscopic uterine nerve ablation – if associated with dysmenorrhoea
    Long-term risks – unknown at present

heavy menstrual blood loss, usually with the passage of fairly large clots, requiring the use of both internal and external protection which needs to be changed every hour or so when the flow is at its worst. Most patients will also give a history of flooding, which usually occurs when they pass urine so that most of this blood is flushed down the toilet; this renders many estimates of menstrual blood loss by observation of tampon staining inaccurate. Patients should have been given a fair trial with medical therapy, particularly prostaglandin synthetase inhibitors and tranexamic acid. Apart from in patients whose menorrhagia is caused by ovulatory disorders, progestogen therapy has never been established as an efficacious treatment, although it is widely used. Many younger patients can be encouraged to take the oral contraceptive or a similar preparation, which will reduce menstrual blood loss in most patients, even though they may not need it for contraception. There is little doubt that endometrial resection is less effective in younger women, and it is worth persevering with medical therapy or possibly going directly to hysterectomy; endometrial resection tends to be more effective in patients in their mid-forties and older.

Endometrial ablation should be advised only when the next logical step would be to advise a hysterectomy and all other methods have failed. The uterus should be smaller than 14 weeks gestational size, with a cavity of 12 cm or less. Many authorities would suggest a slightly lower limit, of 12 weeks and 10 cm[5]. If the patient has large intramural fibroids distorting the cavity, the procedure will be more

---

Key point

Endometrial resection is less effective in younger women.

Key point

Endometrial ablation should only be advised when the next logical step would be to advise a hysterectomy and all other methods have failed.

Preoperative assessment

- Transvaginal ultrasonography
- Endometrial biopsy
- Outpatient hysteroscopy

---

difficult and less successful, but submucous fibroids less than 5 cm in diameter can be removed at the same time as endometrial resection.

The patients should be assessed before operation by transvaginal ultrasonography and endometrial biopsy, preferably associated with outpatient hysteroscopy. Patients with prolapse are better advised to have vaginal hysterectomy and repair of the prolapse, and patients with other conditions such as endometriosis will also require therapy appropriate to the disease. Many patients with painful heavy periods will, not surprisingly, gain no pain relief unless they have some form of procedure to achieve it, such as uterine nerve ablation performed laparoscopically at the same time; if endometriosis is contributing to the dysmenorrhoea, it can be treated by vaporization or ablation via the laparoscope. Although adenomyosis is not a contraindication to endometrial resection, there is little doubt that these patients do not do as well; they often experience quite severe cyclical pain after resection, eventually requiring hysterectomy.

Adequate time must be allowed to explain the procedure and its complications to these patients and I often find it helpful to draw a diagram, at the time of admission for surgery, to explain exactly what is intended. It must be stressed that there is a failure rate of the order of 12%, and that only about a third of patients will become amenorrhoeic and these are usually over 45 years of age. It is also important to explain that complications are possible and may require balloon tamponade or even laparotomy or emergency hysterectomy. It is vital to make the patient understand that this is not a contraceptive procedure and that if she has not been sterilized she must take precautions to avoid pregnancy. She should be offered the possibility of tubal occlusion by laparoscopy at the same time. Patients should be warned that they will have a heavy period after leaving hospital and

> # Key point
>
> There is a failure rate of the order of 12% with endometrial resection, and only about a third of patients will become amenorrhoeic.

that this will become a serosanguineous discharge which can last a few days or even several weeks. They must also be warned that they could have two or three heavy periods during the healing phase, that it takes 6 months for the scar tissue to finally form inside the uterus and that only then can the result be realistically assessed. There is no point in seeing patients for final assessment before that time.

Preoperative preparation

Endometrial thinning

It is essential to have a thin or absent endometrium at the time of the procedure; this can occasionally be arranged if the operation can coincide with a patient's menstrual period, but many of these patients have irregular periods and the logistics of this are by no means easy. The endometrium can be removed by a suction catheter in a similar way to performing a termination of pregnancy, but this often does not give as good a result as one would anticipate, and it also induces a great deal of bleeding.

There is little doubt that the best results are obtained if the endometrium can be prepared by the use of danazol 200 mg twice a day for 6 weeks before the procedure, starting with the onset of menstruation, or by giving LHRH analogues such as Zoladex (ICI Pharmaceuticals, Macclesfield, Cheshire) 3.6 mg as a subcutaneous injection, (Prostap-SR, Lederle, Gosport, UK) or Synarel (Upjohn, Crawley, UK) as a nasal spray in each nostril morning and night. The advantage of injection is that compliance is assured, which may not be the case with the nasal spray in patients in whom it induces severe hot flushes and headaches. Danazol is notorious for its many side-effects but, if the patients can be encouraged to avoid salt-containing food or

> # Key point
>
> It takes 6 months for the scar tissue to form inside the uterus, and only then can the result be realistically assessed.

drink and to drink more pure water, the weight gain is usually minimal and most patients tolerate the side-effects well for the short time that they are on this drug. We have found that the LHRH analogues result in a thinner endometrium and a less active and vascular endometrium, but occasional unwanted side-effects, such as severe cervical stenosis, can also occur with the analogues and are rarely seen with danazol[6].

Analgesia

Most of our patients are admitted for day-case surgery and are in hospital for only a few hours. They are not given any premedication unless they are unusually anxious, and are allowed to return home a few hours after surgery provided they are accompanied by a responsible adult. To avoid unpleasant menstrual cramps after the procedure, 5 ml of bupivacaine is injected as a paracervical block at the completion of surgery.

Prophylactic antibiotics

The operation is performed via the vagina and therefore in a contaminated environment, and the glycine or sorbitol solution, although sterile, is not intended for intravenous use but may enter the bloodstream if there is any extravasation of fluid when the myometrial vessels are transected. For these reasons, it is recommended that patients should receive prophylactic antibiotics. This is slightly controversial, and in over 900 cases when we did not use prophylactic antibiotics we only had one patient with endometritis. Nevertheless endometritis has been reported and is associated with severe morbidity, so this simple prophylactic step is now recommended. We use either Kefzol (Eli Lilly, Basingstoke, UK) or Augmentin (SmithKline Beecham, Brentford, UK).

Equipment

To perform endometrial resection, a rigid hysteroscope is used with a Hopkins rod lens system and fibre optic cable to transmit light from a cold light source. The hysteroscopic resectoscope in common use uses a continuous flow outer sheath (Figure 15.1) to allow optimum visibility – the key to any operative hysteroscopy procedure. Clear irrigating fluid, usually sorbitol or glycine, is circulated under rapid-flow conditions to rinse the uterus of blood and tissue debris that would otherwise obscure the operator's vision. It is essential that isolated inflow and outflow channels run the whole length of the resectoscope so that the fluid flows around the front of the telescope to maintain clear vision at all times. It is also essential that the inflow and outflow tubing is correctly placed according to the direction of the arrows, because the system is not designed for use the other way round. The positions of the outflow ports are extremely important.

Figure 15.1 *Hysteroscopic resectoscope.*

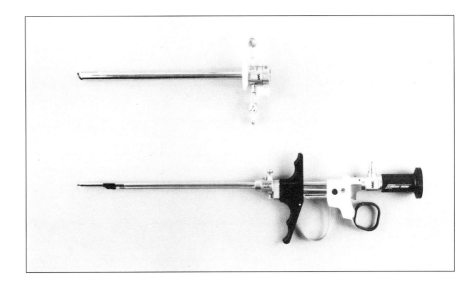

When the outflow holes are provided on only one surface, as with the Storz and Wolf models, the surgeon has to keep rotating the resectoscope, especially when working on the anterior wall, to keep the field of view clear of bubbles. The resectoscopes made by Olympus and Circon ACMI have outer ports that encircle the sheath on the top and bottom surfaces, respectively. This design allows the bubbles that inevitably form during the procedure to be automatically removed and to rise to the top of the uterine cavity, making it unnecessary to shake the end of the resectoscope to clear bubbles from the operator's view[7].

Another difference between the various hysteroscopes is in the angle of vision, which varies widely with the different manufacturers from 0° (Olympus and Storz) to 12° (Circon ACMI), 25° (Wolf) and 30° (Storz and Circon ACMI). The choice is a matter of individual preference, but it is worth testing several different types before purchasing one.

Operative technique

The patient is placed in the lithotomy position and the operating field is cleansed with non-flammable antiseptic solutions and draped in the usual manner. The patient should be asked to void before coming into the operating suite but it is generally not necessary to catheterize patients for this procedure. The resectoscope is assembled with the rollerball in position.

A careful check is made to ensure that there are no air bubbles in the inflow system; the system must be flushed through until all bubbles are removed. This is a vital step, and at all stages of the procedure one member of the operating room staff should be responsible for checking when the fluid container is almost empty and changing containers, to avoid the risk of contamination with air bubbles. It must

---

Safety point

The inflow system must be flushed through until all air bubbles are removed, to remove the risk of air embolism.

---

be realized that, during the procedure of endometrial resection, large myometrial blood vessels are transected and there is instant access to both the arterial and venous systems; if a large air bubble gains access to the circulation an air embolism can occur which is often rapidly fatal. Many deaths have been recorded throughout the world from this complication, and it is the commonest cause of sudden death during this procedure. All theatre personnel must be made aware of this possibility, which can easily be avoided by diligence.

The cervix is grasped by two vulsellum forceps attached to the anterior lip, and the uterine cavity measured with the uterine sound to check that it does not exceed 12 cm. The cervix is carefully dilated to a diameter just in excess of the diameter of the resectoscope and, with the fluid running, the resectoscope is introduced to inspect the inside of the cavity. The operator should check on the position of the tubal orifices and note any anatomical abnormalities, such as an intrauterine septum or submucous fibroid, that may have gone undetected in the preoperative work-up.

Common reasons for a poor view at hysteroscopy

- Fogging of video equipment due to temperature differential or dampness
- Insufficient inflow pressure
- Kinking of suction or irrigation tubing
- Blockage of outflow tubes by tissue debris

No energy source should be activated unless there is an absolutely clear view, and if the view is obscured by blood or tissue debris the reason for this must be sought and rectified before proceeding to any electrosurgery. (There may be insufficient pressure or flow on the inflow side, due to either kinking of the tube or incorrect diameter of delivery tubes, or the outflow system may be blocked by tissue debris.) Once a clear view is obtained and the electrosurgical generator is

Safety point

It is essential to obtain a clear view of the uterine cavity before proceeding to electrosurgery.

activated and the current mode and strength selected, the rollerball is placed in the cornual area and the foot pedal depressed as the rollerball is moved towards the operator. The rollerball should always be pulled towards the operator and never pushed forward whilst the current is on.

The cornual region is the thinnest part of the uterus (possibly only a few millimetres thick) and rollerball coagulation can easily damage tissue up to 3 mm in depth[8] (Figure 15.2). Once the cornual area is coagulated with three or four radial strokes coming down towards the operator for about 1–2 cm (A in Figure 15.2), the rollerball is rolled across the fundus (B) to the other cornual area where a similar procedure takes place (A). When starting hysteroscopic electrosurgery, it is safer to test the tissue effect of the rollerball at a mid-point in the fundal region where the uterus is at its thickest, to make sure that the power density of the electrical energy is not too fierce. Great caution should be exercised in the cornual region because of its thinness; many cases have been recorded where

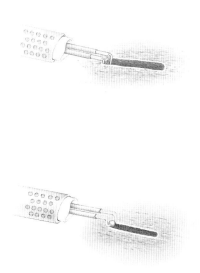
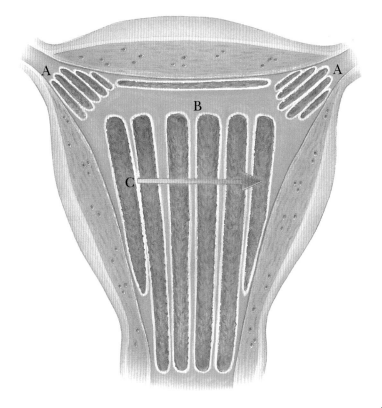

Figure 15.2 *Systematic approach to endometrial resection commencing with rollerball ablation of the cornual and fundal regions.*

Safety point

The rollerball should always be pulled towards the operator and **never** pushed forward while the current is on.

coagulative necrosis has occurred and the cornual area has later perforated during the procedure merely due to the hydrostatic pressure of the irrigating fluid on the weakened tissue.

Once careful coagulation of both cornua has been achieved the rollerball is changed for a resectoscope loop, which is extended to its full length, sunk into the myometrium to its full depth and pulled back towards the end of the hysteroscope at the same time withdrawing the hysteroscope to remove an endometrial strip down to the level of the internal os. It is vital to raise the loop gradually to the surface as one approaches the internal os because deep resection at this level will almost certainly result in extremely heavy bleeding if branches of the lateral cervical arteries are unintentionally transected. At the end of each sweep, the entire strip is removed on the end of the resectoscope loop, and as the resectoscope is withdrawn from the cervix an assistant picks up the strip and places it on a gauze swab. The advantage of this technique is that there is no tissue debris left inside the uterus to obscure the operator's vision, and by allowing the fluids to empty at the end of each sweep there is no possibility of fluid overload developing. We have used this technique on more than 1000 patients without a single episode of fluid overload. It also has the advantage of allowing the histologist to orientate the specimen to obtain an accurate measure of endometrial thickness and activity, and to select particular areas to take specimens from.

The depth of penetration is to a large extent dependent on the size of loop used and we have found that results are just as good with a 7 mm loop as with the more widely used 9 mm loop. The cross-striations of the myometrial muscle can be easily recognized and differentiated from endometrium, and it is important to go down to that level, but on no account should the operator attempt a repeat pass because the combined penetration would be much too deep and could result in perforation.

As soon as the hysteroscopic view becomes panoramic the internal os has been reached and resection should not continue beneath this level, not only because of the risk of damage to the cervical arteries but because it also increases the risk of subsequent cervical stenosis and haematometra.

Instead of using this technique, some surgeons chip away at the endometrium. They can, of course, achieve the same result, but need to evacuate all the tissue debris periodically. Also because of the length

> # Safety point
>
> A repeat pass of the resectoscope should **never** be made over the tissue once the fibres of the myometrium have been seen.

of time that the irrigating fluid is kept inside the uterus, it is more likely that fluid overload will occur. A careful watch must be kept on the input and the output: a nurse should be measuring this all the time. The surgeon must be warned if the deficit is over 1 litre, when it may be necessary to stop the procedure or at least warn the anaesthetist to watch for signs of fluid overload and possibly administer diuretics. If the fluid deficit exceeds $1^1/_2$ litres the surgery should be completed as quickly as possible, and if it exceeds 2 litres, severe hyponatraemia and other metabolic disturbances are highly likely and surgery should be stopped immediately. At the end of the procedure bupivacaine hydrochloride is injected as a paracervical block at 7 o'clock and 4 o'clock, taking care to check that a vessel has not been inadvertently entered by withdrawing on the syringe before injecting the local anaesthetic.

Some surgeons prefer to complete the procedure by superficially coagulating the area already resected, and this does allow any large vessels to be sealed by thermocoagulation. By lowering the inflow these vessels can be easily identified, but in practice this can merely be alarming: most of these vessels will seal using the body's own haemostatic mechanisms. Only vessels that are spurting at the normal intrauterine pressure used for the operating procedure require to be sealed with the rollerball, and if this is not possible and the patient is bleeding heavily at the end of the procedure a 30 ml balloon catheter should be inserted and the balloon inflated to allow tamponade of the bleeding blood vessels. This is rarely necessary, and usually by the time the nursing staff have assembled the necessary equipment the bleeding has stopped, but if it is the patient should not be discharged as a day-case but should stay in hospital overnight and have the catheter removed the following morning. Prophylactic antibiotics should certainly be used in this situation.

Conclusion

Electrosurgical endometrial resection looks easy to the uninitiated when an expert performs it. It is, however, associated with more complications than any other procedure in the whole field of endoscopic surgery. For this reason, instruction in the physics associated with electrosurgery and the hydrodynamics inherent in the

Key point

Only vessels that are actively bleeding at normal operative intrauterine pressure will need specific measures to achieve haemostasis. If bleeding is not stopped by rollerball, tamponade can be achieved with a 30 ml balloon Foley catheter.

fluid systems used to ensure a good clear view is essential before a surgeon embarks on these procedures. Electrical energy should never be activated unless the surgeon can clearly see the field of operation, and the rollerball or wire loop must always be pulled towards the operator, and *never* activated when it is pushed away from the operator.

The surgeon should be absolutely familiar with the hysteroscopic appearance of normal and abnormal uteri and should have performed at least 50 diagnostic hysteroscopies before embarking on an operative procedure. Various simulators and uterine models (see Chapter 3) should then be used: it is possible to use both lasers and electrosurgery with these models and the tissue effects simulated are very close to those encountered during surgery, although there is of course no bleeding. The next step is to use other simulators, such as a potato with a central cylinder bored out of it with an apple corer immersed in a solution of glycine. Following this, a number of procedures should be performed on uteri that have been removed from patients who have had a hysterectomy and, finally, on a series of patients who have given their consent for an endometrial resection to be performed before the uterus is removed at hysterectomy so that the surgeon can learn this technique. The initial live procedures should be carried out under the supervision of someone who is experienced in these techniques, and it is better to begin with rollerball coagulation alone until experience is achieved. If at any stage of the procedure the view is obscured, the procedure should be stopped until this is corrected. If, at any time there is a fluid deficit of more than $1^1/_2$ litres the surgery should either be finished rapidly or stopped and, if at any time the hysteroscopist sees a view similar to that obtained at laparoscopy, a perforation has occurred and the procedure should be immediately

Safety point

Electrical energy should never be activated unless the surgeon can clearly see the field of operation and the rollerball or wire loop must always be pulled towards the operator and **never** activated when it is pushed away from the operator.

abandoned and either laparoscopy or laparotomy undertaken. Laparoscopy will reveal the extent of the perforation and the amount of bleeding but cannot reliably check the bowel for any sign of damage. Laparotomy will allow a careful inspection of bowel, and if there is any injury a wide excision of the area involved should be undertaken by a surgical colleague because damage can occur up to 5 cm from the site of an electrical injury. Even if bowel perforation is not discovered the patient must be kept in hospital for at least 3 days and, if she shows signs of increasing pain or develops a temperature, laparotomy will be necessary to repair the bowel injury that is almost certain to be the cause.

Transcervical resection of the endometrium is useful for patients with menorrhagia or submucous fibroids. Although it looks simple to perform, it is extremely difficult and requires a learning curve of at least 50 operations before the operator can be said to be competent in its performance. Complications can occur very quickly and can be associated with severe morbidity, and are occasionally fatal.

Nevertheless, when performed well by an experienced operator, it does appear to be safe with good short-term results of about 90% effectiveness. We have found in a 5 year follow-up that the failure rate stabilizes after about $2^{1}/_{2}$ years and remains constant at 75% thereafter. This figure shows that three quarters of patients can avoid hysterectomy by a simple day-case procedure, and our patients are advised to return to work and full activity within 48 h.

Summary

Approximately 60% of women with menorrhagia severe enough to consider hysterectomy are suitable for treatment by endometrial resection. Pre–operative assessment including transvaginal ultrasonography, endometrial biopsy and outpatient hysteroscopy will identify those women who have a uterus of less than 14 weeks gestational size and a cavity less than 12 cm. Operative results are best if the endometrium is absent or thin at the time of the procedure, a situation that is achieved by either operating in the menstrual phase or pre–treating the patient with Danazol or GnRH analogues. The majority of procedures are done as day–case operations, without pre–medication, returning home with a responsible adult. A para–cervical block is used to ease post–operative pain and prophylactic antibiotics are given intra–operatively. A clear view of the uterine cavity should be obtained before commencing electrosurgery. A rollerball is used to effect coagulation of both uterine cornua and a resectoscopic loop is used for the rest of the cavity. Entire strips of endometrium should be removed at the end of each sweep, permitting fluids to drain from the cavity thus reducing the risk of fluid overload. At least 50 operations should be performed before an operator can be considered to be competent. A competent surgeon should expect to have a 90% short–term effectiveness in reducing the degree of menorrhagia falling to 75% five years post–operatively.

References

1. Goldrath MH, Fuller TA, Segal S (1981) Laser photovaporisation of endometrium for the treatment of menorrhagia. *Am J Obstet Gynecol* **140**: 14–19.
2. Neuwirth RS (1978) A new technique for and addition experience with hysteroscopic resection of submucous fibroids. *Am J Obstet Gynecol* **131**: 91–4.
3. DeCherney AH, Polan ML (1983) Hysteroscopic management of intrauterine lesion and intractable uterine bleeding. *Obstet Gynecol* **61**: 392–7.
4. Rutherford AJ, Glass MR, Wells M (1991) Patient selection for endometrial resection. *Br J Obstet Gynaecol* **98**: 228–30.
5. Broadbent JAM, Magos AL (1993) Transcervical resection of the endometrium. In: Sutton C, Diamond M (eds) *Endoscopic Surgery for Gynaecologists*. WB Saunders, London, pp. 294–306.
6. Sutton CJG, Ewen SP (1994) Thinning the endometrium prior to endometrial ablation: is it worthwhile? *Br J Obstet Gynaecol* **101** (Suppl. 10): 10–12.
7. Brooks PG (1990) Resectoscopes for the gynaecologist. *Contemp Obstet Gynaecol* 51–6.
8. Duffy S, Reid PC, Smith JH, Sharp F (1991) Studies of uterine electrosurgery. *Obstet Gynecol* **78**: 213–20.

Chapter 16
Endometrial Laser Ablation
R. Garry

Introduction

This chapter describes the safe performance of endometrial ablation using an Nd-YAG laser. The equipment required is described in some detail, and the use of pretreatment regimens to thin the endometrium before surgery is discussed. A detailed account of the operative procedure and postoperative care is also included, with a critical review of the results of this surgery and a brief review of the common complications.

Management of dysfunctional uterine bleeding

The concept of precisely removing only diseased or dysfunctional tissue and conserving as much healthy tissue as possible is good surgical practice. Defining dysplastic epithelium and accurately removing only the abnormal tissue under colposcopic control has almost completely replaced the need for hysterectomy in the management of abnormal cervical cytology.

The causes of dysfunctional uterine bleeding (DUB) are not completely known. It remains a major indication for hysterectomy. It is estimated that more than 50% of the 70 000 hysterectomies done in the UK each year are performed to manage excessive menstrual bleeding in the absence of structural pathology.

It has long seemed an attractive concept that DUB should be managed by removing only the dysfunctional endometrium and conserving the healthy remainder of the uterus. The problem with this concept is that the endometrium is shed physiologically each month and has amazing powers of regeneration. Most locally applied destructive agents merely slough off the superficial endometrium, which can then regenerate from the persisting glands located deep in the endometrium. If excess menstrual bleeding is to be prevented in a permanent way, it is essential to remove the whole thickness of the endometrium and the superficial layers of the myometrium. Only in this way will the basal glands be removed and regrowth of the endometrium prevented.

The first clinically useful method of removing the endometrium was a technique of ablation using an Nd-YAG laser described by Milton Goldrath in 1981. The principle of this approach is that Nd-YAG laser energy passes unabsorbed through clear fluids, including tissue fluids, but coagulates tissue proteins by a thermal effect. Nd-YAG laser energy passes a fairly constant depth into tissues such as the endometrium and destroys a consistent 4–5 mm of tissue. The laser energy can be easily transmitted to the treatment site down flexible quartz fibres and will pass unaffected through the clear fluids used to distend the uterine cavity. The clinical advantages are summarized below.

Properties of the Nd-YAG laser energy

- Passes down flexible fibre
- Passes unabsorbed through clear fluids
- Photovaporizes the endometrium
- Penetrates tissue for 5 mm

Equipment

Nd-YAG laser

The clinical effect at tissue is dependent on the power delivered, the surface area of the delivery fibre and the duration of application.

The higher the power applied, the deeper the zone of destruction produced or the faster the fibre can be drawn over the surface to produce a constant effect. I have found high laser powers important and prefer to have a 100 W laser set to deliver 80 W of power at tissue. Lower power lasers require substantially longer treatment times.

The standard size fibre for endometrial laser ablation (ELA) is only 600 μm in diameter. This small surface area produces a high power density. Larger diameter fibres, which would appear to be very desirable to complete the surgery more quickly, in fact dissipate the available energy over a larger area, thereby reducing the power density, so that the fibre must be pulled more slowly over the endometrium. This prolongs the treatment time and negates any possible advantage of using a larger diameter fibre.

The fibre used for ELA must be a simple quartz fibre. Elaborate tips should not be used: they are of no advantage and, if the tips are inadvertently cooled by coaxial gas, they may be lethal.

Hysteroscopes

When Goldrath first described the technique[1], there was no suitable hysteroscope for operative laser surgery. The hysteroscope he used had only an operating channel and a single fluid channel. Fluid could be instilled into the cavity, but there was no way in which it could leave the cavity. To overcome this design fault, he initially recommended that the cervix be hyperdilated so that fluid could escape around the hysteroscope barrel.

Subsequently, outflow channels for fluid egress have been added to operating hysteroscopes. It is now appreciated that the best operating conditions are obtained with a continuous flow system containing discrete channels for fluid inflow and outflow (Figure 16.1). The ideal hysteroscope should have a smooth outside barrel of circular cross-section to fit snugly in the dilated cervical canal. A good fit

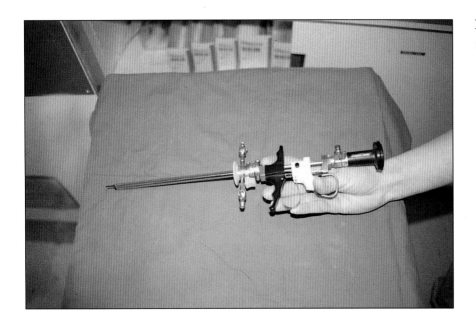

Figure 16.1 *Continuous flow hysteroscope.*

between the hysteroscope and the cervix will prevent leakage of fluid from the cavity and contain all the fluid in a closed system.

Almost all workers in this field prefer to use a rigid hysteroscope with a high-quality Hopkins rod lens system. A 4 or 5 mm diameter telescope will give a good quality image and leave sufficient room to incorporate fluid and operating channels into an overall diameter compatible with standard cervical dilatation techniques.

Flexible hysteroscopes are available and have been used for operative hysteroscopy most notably by Cornier[2] in Paris. These usually have a narrower diameter, are softer and can be more easily inserted into the uterine cavity under direct vision. This property is of particular value in patients with a sharply retroverted uterus and in patients with a narrow or stenosed cervical canal. The image is, however, usually smaller and less sharp compared with that obtained with a rigid hysteroscope. Flexible hysteroscopes are also more expensive than the rigid type.

Uterine distension systems

In the natural state, the uterine cavity is dark and only a potential space with the anterior and posterior walls in approximation. To ensure a clear view of the cavity, good quality cold light must be directed down a flexible fibre into a cavity distended with either gas or an optically clear fluid under pressure.

The minimum pressure required to distend the cavity is 40–50 mmHg, which can be achieved by suspending a bag 1 m above the patient. The infusion pressure can be altered by varying the height of the bag or by applying an inflatable cuff around a soft fluid bag. Fluid may also be infused using peristaltic pumps, which can be either simple pumps or pressure-regulated pumps. Simple pumps produce a constant flow but, if the outflow resistance varies, the pressure inside the uterine cavity may vary and, if it rises, excess fluid absorption may be a problem. Automatic pressure pumps are therefore safer and to be preferred.

Distension media

Almost all workers use a fluid distension medium for endometrial ablation. The exception is Adolf Gallinat, who believes that carbon dioxide gas, under carefully controlled conditions, provides a safer but still effective distension medium[3]. Much smoke is generated with ablation in gas, and this rapidly obscures vision unless continuously removed.

Clear fluids, however, provide excellent vision. The choice of fluid is dependent on the nature of the energy source. When electrical energy is used, a solution without electrolytes is required. Such a solution does nothing for the quality of the image but increases the dangers of the procedure if absorbed in excess; circulatory failure, hyponatraemia, metabolic disturbances, cerebral oedema, coma and even death may result. The use of such fluids is, however, mandatory when monopolar electricity is used because the current is dissipated and the equipment does not work in an electrolyte-containing medium, which conducts electricity.

No such constraints apply when using laser energy, and the safest and most convenient fluid such as normal saline or Hartmann's solution may be used. Such solutions are more physiological and, although they can still provoke fluid overload if absorbed in excess, they do not cause electrolyte or metabolic problems and are therefore to be preferred.

Tissue effects of the Nd-YAG laser

As the laser energy collides with a tissue, it generates heat. When the tissue temperature reaches more than 55 °C protein is denatured and coagulated, and when it reaches 100 °C intracellular water boils and cell membranes are destroyed. At temperatures above 150 °C carbonization occurs, and above 300 °C, tissue vaporization occurs. At the tip of the laser fibre temperature rise is great and tissue vaporization occurs, producing the characteristic furrow. Beneath this zone of vaporization is a thin zone of charring where the temperature rise was not so great, and beneath the char is a zone of tissue coagulation and protein denaturization which, in the endometrium, extends for about 4–5 mm beneath the zone of vaporization (Figure 16.2).

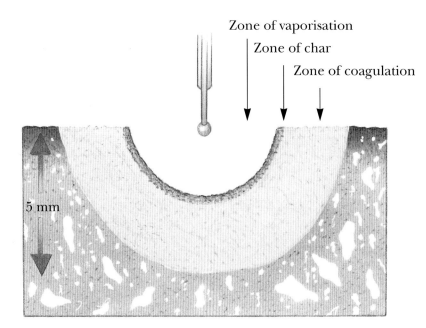

Zone of vaporisation

Zone of char

Zone of coagulation

5 mm

Figure 16.2 *Nd-YAG laser destruction.*

Preoperative endometrial thinning

The endometrium varies in thickness during the menstrual cycle and, in the late secretory phase, may be 8–10 mm thick. As Nd-YAG laser energy penetrates only 5 mm into tissue, attempted ablation at this stage of the cycle is doomed to failure because the basal glands in the superficial myometrium will not be affected. It is possible to schedule surgery to occur early in the menstrual cycle, but it is practically easier to artificially ensure that the endometrium is always as thin as possible at the time of ablation by pretreatment (Figure 16.3).

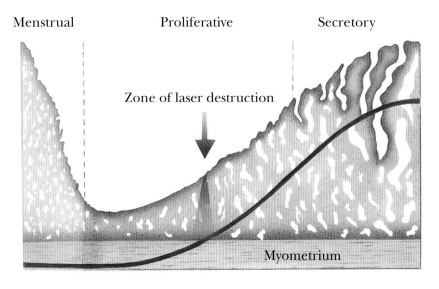

Menstrual   Proliferative   Secretory

Zone of laser destruction

Myometrium

Figure 16.3 *Composite diagram of endometrium throughout the menstrual cycle.*

The preparation first suggested by Goldrath to thin the endometrium was danazol in a dose of 600–800 mg daily for 3–6 weeks. A recent trial comparing this drug with the GnRH analogue goserelin (Zoladex, Zeneca Pharmaceuticals, Macclesfield, UK) demonstrated that goserelin produced a thinner endometrium and a smaller uterine cavity volume. The better preparation was associated with a 25% reduction in treatment time. Goserelin is particularly indicated in patients with submucous fibroids and with larger uteri.

Technique

Endometrial laser ablation is usually performed under general anaesthesia but may easily be performed under regional or local anaesthesia if preferred.

The patient is placed in the lithotomy position with the legs carefully supported and then cleaned and draped in the standard manner. Preoperative shaving and bladder catheterization are not required. A tenaculum is placed on the anterior lip of the cervix and then the cervix is dilated to a diameter just sufficient to accommodate the hysteroscope. The aim is to secure a watertight seal between the hysteroscope and the cervix. An operating hysteroscope is then inserted through the cervix under direct vision. A continuous flow of 0.9% saline is established at a pressure between 50 and 80 mmHg and the fluid escaping from the outflow channel of the hysteroscope is collected and carefully measured at repeated intervals. The most modern hysteroscope pumping systems are able to measure the inflow and outflow volumes and continuously compute the fluid deficit.

The hysteroscope should be connected to a high-intensity light source by a good quality quartz fibre cable. A single-chip or three-chip CCD video camera and monitor are essential. To maintain crystal clear vision throughout the procedure, it is essential that the surgeon understands the fluid mechanics inside the uterine cavity. The subendometrial blood vessels are inevitably disrupted during any hysteroscopic procedure and, if the bleeding is not controlled, will inevitably obscure vision. Raising the intrauterine pressure sufficiently in a closed system will, however, compress and tamponade the vessels and prevent such bleeding. In a well conducted case, no bleeding should occur at any stage. Unfortunately, if the pressure in the cavity is raised too high, fluid will be forced into the disrupted blood vessels and fluid overload may occur. The aim in hysteroscopic surgery is to distend the uterine cavity with sufficient pressure to prevent bleeding but with a pressure low enough to avoid forcing fluid into the patient's vascular system. This 'titration' can be most easily performed with pressure-controlled pumps.

The shape and appearance of the cavity and the endometrial surface are carefully observed, looking particularly for any areas suggestive of malignant or premalignant change. If an endometrial sample has not been obtained previously, one or more hysteroscopically directed biopsies should be taken.

Protective goggles should be worn by everyone in the operating theatre, and warning signs illuminated at every entry to the operating room. When the laser is activated, entry to the room is prohibited to everyone not wearing appropriate eye protection.

Only when everything is ready and an optimum view of the endometrium is present is the laser activated at a power of 80 W. Beginning usually at the right tubal ostium, the laser fibre is applied to the surface, activated and then drawn back towards the cervix in such a way as to produce a furrow through the thickness of the endometrium. A series of such parallel furrows are then produced until the whole of the peritubal area is ablated. The procedure is repeated around the left ostial area and then areas on the fundus and anterior and posterior uterine wall are treated systematically until the whole cavity down to the level of the internal os is treated (Figure 16.4).

To achieve efficient ablation, it is essential to move the hysteroscope through an arc to keep the fibre in contact with the endometrium as it is being withdrawn. The fibre is pulled out using the right hand and the hysteroscope is held in the left hand. Beginners greatly underestimate the length of arc the left hand must move through to keep the fibre on the surface. Remember that the hysteroscope is pivoted very near its distal end and so a considerable amount of movement at the proximal end is required to move the tip through a very small arc (Figure 16.5).

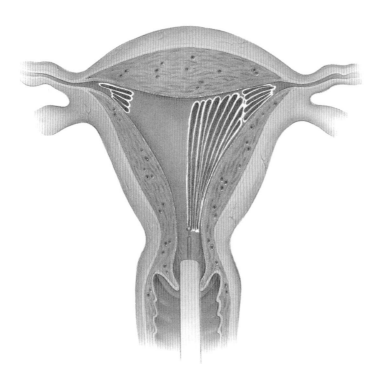

Figure 16.4 *Systematic ablation of the uterine cavity.*

Figure 16.5 *Movement of the hysteroscope.*

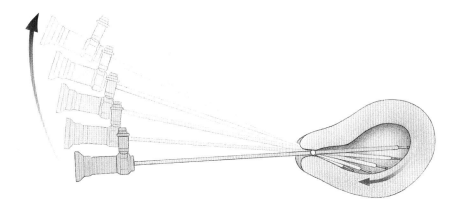

The tip of the fibre glows red because there is a second HeNe laser built into the system. This glowing tip should always be visible and, if it is, the laser fibre *must* be in the uterine cavity. There are three safety rules (summarized below). The third, is important because it will ensure that the laser can never perforate the uterus while it is activated. Using such a system, we have not sustained a uterine perforation in more than 1200 cases.

The three golden rules of safety

- Only fire the laser when the fibre tip is seen glowing
- Only fire the laser when the fibre is moving
- Only fire the laser when the fibre is being drawn towards the operator

Postoperative care

The procedure usually takes between 15 and 30 min to complete. When the whole cavity has been satisfactorily ablated, which should have been completed without bleeding or interruption to remove chips of endometrium, etc., the laser is turned off and the instruments are removed. A paracervical block with 1% bupivacaine (10 ml may be injected at both 9 o'clock and 3 o'clock). This has been shown to reduce immediate postoperative pain and the need for opiate analgesia. The patient usually recovers within a few hours and is fit to leave hospital the same day.

Patients should be advised that menstrual-like discomfort is to be anticipated and should be sent home with some simple analgesics and an information booklet. The patient (and her general practitioner) should be warned to anticipate a serosanguineous loss, rather like lochia, which can persist for up to 6 weeks. This is seldom infected and rarely requires antibiotics.

Surgical outcome and residual symptoms

The results of our first 600 consecutive ELAs performed on 524 women have recently been reviewed. The mean operating time was 25 min and the average amount of fluid deficit was 603 ml. There was no major morbidity and no case of perforation of the uterus with the laser. No case required immediate laparoscopy, laparotomy or hysterectomy. Neither was there a single case of haemorrhage or requiring emergency blood transfusion.

Postal questionnaires were returned by 501 of the 524 women (96%). The mean length of follow-up was 15 months. A second procedure was required by 76 women of whom one had a third ablation. At the time of review, 29 (6.1%) had subsequently undergone a hysterectomy and this percentage is slowly rising. A total of 135 (29%) developed complete amenorrhoea. Of the remainder who were still menstruating after the treatment, 90% described a profound reduction in the volume of bleeding. Dysmenorrhoea responded less well; although 57% of those with dysmenorrhoea felt that the pain was improved by the operation, 31% felt that it was unimproved and 7.9% felt that it was worse. Only six (3.9%) developed pain for the first time after the ablation.

The patients described the overall results as excellent in 52% of cases, good in 31% and disappointing or a failure in 16.6%. The younger the patient at the time of treatment, the more likely the treatment was to deal completely with the patient's symptoms. Two pregnancies occurred after the ablation. One was terminated at 12 weeks and the other was delivered satisfactorily at term without obvious problem.

Complications

Our experience suggests that ELA is a relatively safe procedure with few complications. There are papers in the literature to warn of the possible risks. Three cases of uterine perforation have been reported[4]. Significant intraoperative haemorrhage is unlikely, but major postoperative bleeding remains a possibility. Significant quantities of necrotic material remain in the uterine cavity and could provide a focus for infection. I recommend the use of a single-administration peroperative broad-spectrum antibiotic to minimize this risk.

The first ELA was performed in 1979. Long-term follow-up data are not yet available, and it is essential that audit of these procedures should continue. We need to have a clear idea of the rate of late failures of these treatments. We also have to maintain vigilant follow-up to determine the risk of subsequent uterine malignancy.

Conclusion

The evidence available to date suggest that ELA is an effective and safe procedure, which may be of benefit to many patients suffering from dysfunctional uterine bleeding.

Summary

Endometrial laser ablation is a safe and effective method of treating dysfunctional uterine bleeding by the hysteroscopic technique. Pre-treatment with with GnRH analogues will lead to the reduction of endometrial thickness to less than 5mm permitting full thickness tissue destruction. If GnRH analogues are not administered, the procedure should be performed in the early proliferative phase of the menstrual cycle. Continuous flow of 0.9% saline or Hartmann's solution is used to distend the uterine cavity leading to less risk of electrolyte and metabolic disturbances than less physiological fluids. Typically, the duration of the procedure is 15–30 minutes, and a paracervical block is used to reduce the severity of immediate post–operative pain, permitting the patient to leave hospital on the same day. Intra–operative antibiotics are advised. Between 50–80% of patients report high rates of satisfaction with the procedure, a failure rate of 16.5% being reported.

References

1. Goldrath MH, Fuller TA, Segal S (1981) Laser photovaporization of endometrium for the treatment of menorrhagia. *Am J Obstet Gynecol* **140**: 14–19.
2. Cornier E (1986) Fibro-hysteroscopique ambulatoire des metrorragies rebelles par laser Nd:YAG. *J Gynecol Obstet Biol Reprod* **15**: 661–4.
3. Gallinat A, Lueken RR, Moller CP (1989) The use of the Nd-YAG laser in gynecological endoscopy. Laser brief 14, Medizintechnik, Munich.
4. Perry CP, Daniell JG, Gimpleson RJ (1990) Bowel injury from Nd YAG endometrial ablation. *J Gynecol Surg* **6**: 199–203.

Bibliography

Baggish MS, Baltoyannis P (1988) New techniques for laser ablation of the endometrium in high risk patients. *Am J Obstet Gynecol* **159**: 287–92.

Baggish MS, Daniell JF (1989) Death caused by air embolism associated with neodymium yttrium aluminum garnet laser surgery and artificial sapphire tips. *Am J Obstet Gynecol* **161**: 877–9.

Dallay D, Tissot H, Portal F (1992) Endometrectomie par hysterofibroscopie laser YAG. *J Gynecol Obstet Biol Reprod* **21**: 431–5.

Garry R, Erian J, Grochmal SAL (1991) A multi-centre collaborative study into the treatment of menorrhagia by Nd-YAG laser ablation of the endometrium. *Br J Obstet Gynaecol* **98**: 357–62.

Garry R, Mooney P, Hasham F, Kokri M (1992) A uterine distension system to prevent fluid absorption during Nd-YAG laser endometrial laser ablation. *Gynaecol Endosc* **1**: 23–7.

Hasham F, Garry R, Kokri MS, Mooney P (1992) Fluid absorption during laser ablation of the endometrium in the treatment of menorrhagia. *Br J Anaesth* **68**: 151–4.

Loffer FD (1987) Hysteroscopic endometrial ablation with Nd-YAG laser in the treatment of menorrhagia. *J Reprod Med* **31**: 148–50.

Lomano JM (1988) Photocoagulation of the endometrium with Nd-YAG laser in the treatment of menorrhagia. *J Reprod Med* **31**: 148–50.

Magos AL, Bauman R, Lockwood GM, Turnbull AC (1991) Experience with the first 250 endometrial resections for menorrhagia. *Lancet* **377**: 1074–8.

Perry CP, Daniell JF, Gimpleson RJ (1990) Bowel injury from Nd-YAG endometrial ablation. *J Gynecol Surg* **6**: 199–203.

Chapter 17

Hysteroscopic Treatment of Submucous Fibroids

J. G. Donnez, R. Polet, M. Smets, S. Bassil
and M. Nisolle

Introduction

This chapter proposes a truly minimally invasive method of treating uterine fibroids using a fibre optic laser delivery system at hysteroscopy. The case is made for the use of lasers in preference to electrosurgical resectoscopes. A clear step–by–step guide to the operation procedures is provided together with an extensive audit of operation outcomes.

Advantages of lasers over resectoscopes

Both the electrical current of the resectoscope and the energy of the Nd-YAG laser are effective tools for removing submucous fibroids. The fact that the resectoscope is a unipolar electrical instrument is a possible disadvantage. There is the potential for damaging the bowel and the bladder with the current transmitted through the uterine wall with the cutting loop. In addition, there is the risk of bleeding if major uterine vessels are transected by cutting too deeply into the uterine wall[1–3]. On the other hand, the resectoscope has an advantage over the laser in that the equipment is readily available in most operating rooms as it is the same equipment used for urological procedures. Another advantage is that the resectoscope does not require the major capital investment needed for a laser. However, laser energy is a more precise method of tissue destruction[4].

Nd-YAG laser energy, in particular, has several physical properties which make it particularly suitable for transhysteroscopic use[5]. Transmission of the laser energy into the uterine cavity is carried out through flexible quartz fibres; it travels readily in liquid medium and is absorbed by the proteins of the tissue with which the beam comes into contact. The interaction of the laser with the tissue takes place in the optical zone, the depth of which is relatively dependent on the level of energy applied to the tissue and the duration of exposure. The depth of this area is controlled[6–8] to be around 4–6 mm; this physical quality can be applied for transhysteroscopic myomectomy and myolysis[9-10].

The Nd-YAG laser has been successfully used for endometrial ablation, hysteroscopic endometrial[5,7,8,11], synechiae[12], intrauterine septum[13] and endometrial polyps.

Submucous myomas are associated with infertility and menorrhagia, although the involvement of fibroids in infertility is still unclear.

The nature and the extent of the operation to be performed takes into account the complaint, the type of submucous fibroid and the desire of the patient to retain fertility.

Physical properties of the Nd-YAG laser that facilitate hysteroscopic use

- Laser energy is transmitted through flexible quartz fibres
- Laser energy travels readily in liquid medium
- Laser energy is absorbed by the proteins of the tissue with which the beam comes into contact
- The interaction of the laser with the tissue takes place in the optical zone
- The depth of tissue destruction depends on the level of energy applied and the duration of exposure
- The depth of this area is constant at around 4–6 mm

Instruments and equipment

The fibre used to carry the laser light consists of quartz, surrounded by a thin plastic jacket, beyond which the tip of the fibre extends for several millimetres. The fibre is gas-sterilized or wiped with alcohol or Cidex (Surgikos, Livingston, UK) before use.

The deflecting arm is not of particular value, but allows the fibre to be stabilized. New instruments are now available in which the telescope is inserted into two sheaths of varying diameter: one for inflow and the other for outflow. This resembles the classic resectoscope[14] and permits the constant cleaning of the uterine cavity. This system has been called the continuous-flow hysteroscope. We provide constant uterine distension by attaching one 3000 ml plastic bag of 1.5% glycine or saline solution to the inflow tubing. The bag is then wrapped in a pressure infusion cuff, similar to that used to infuse blood under pressure, and the tube is connected to the hysteroscope. Since continuous flow hysteroscopy has been used, overload fluid has not occurred. This very simple system, which does not require any sophisticated and expensive pumps, allows the surgeon to perform hysteroscopic surgery in optimal conditions.

A Sharplan 2100 apparatus (Sharplan, Tel-Aviv, Israel; Figure 17.1) is used for generating the laser. A power output of 80 W is selected.

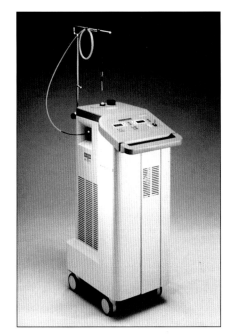

Figure 17.1 *Sharplan Nd-YAG laser (courtesy of Litechnica Ltd., Heston, UK).*

Diagnosis

The diagnosis of intracavitary fibroids is always confirmed by hysterography and outpatient hysteroscopy with directed endometrial biopsy. Submucous fibroids are classified as listed below (according to hysterosalpingography findings).

Classification of submucous fibroids

1. Submucous fibroids whose greatest diameter is located inside the uterine cavity (Figure 17.2a)
2. Submucous fibroids whose greatest diameter is located in the myometrium (Figure 17.2b)
3. Multiple (more than two) submucous fibroids (myofibromatous uterus with submucous fibroids and intramural fibroids) diagnosed by hysterography and echography (Figure 17.2c)

The patients are considered suitable for hysteroscopic surgery only if the histological sampling fails to reveal any malignant or highly suspicious endometrial condition.

All cases suitable for hysteroscopic treatment are prepared with gonadotrophin-releasing hormone (GnRH) analogues, to decrease the size of the uterine cavity and the size of the fibroid to be treated, and to restore a satisfactory preoperative level of haemoglobin. In addition, the extreme endometrial atrophy clears the operative field and facilitates the operative procedure; it is therefore faster, involves fewer peroperative complications and probably decreases the risk of recurrence.

We use a biodegradable GnRH analogue (Zoladex implant, Zeneca Pharmaceuticals, Macclesfield, UK). The implant is injected

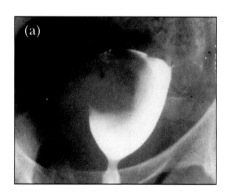
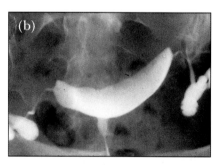
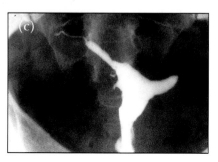

Figure 17.2 *Hysterographic classification of submucous fibroids, according to Donnez and Nisolle: (a) submucous fibroid whose greatest diameter is inside the uterine cavity, (b) submucous fibroid whose greatest diameter is inside the uterine wall, (c) multiple submucosal myomas (reproduced with permission from Sutton & Diamond (eds)* Endoscopic Surgery for Gynaecologists, *W. B. Saunders & Co. Ltd, London, 1992).*

> # Key point
>
> All patients receive preoperative treatment with GnRH analogues.

subcutaneously at the end of the luteal phase to curtail the initial gonadotrophin stimulation phase and the associated rise in oestrogen. One implant is administered at each of weeks 0, 4 and 8. Hysteroscopic myomectomy is carried out at week 8. The day before surgery, repeat hysterography enables us to calculate the reduction in area of the uterine cavity and of the fibroid using the short-line multipurpose test system described by Weibel, allowing assessment of the GnRH analogue treatment[9,10].

We shall describe here our observations from 376 women whose mean age was 33 years (range 23–43 years) who were all suffering from symptomatic submucous fibroids. After the initial stimulation of oestrogen secretion, GnRH agonist administration reduced oestrogen levels to the postmenopausal range (15 ± 6 pg/ml). Luteinizing hormone and follicle-stimulating hormone levels were significantly suppressed following 2 weeks of treatment. Recovery of ovarian secretion occurred an average of 4–5 weeks after the last injection[10].

Using the method previously described, the reduction in area of large submucous fibroids was calculated. When more than one fibroid was present, only the largest was evaluated. In all but four patients, the fibroid area decreased by an average of 38% (range 4–95%)[15]. The fibroid area was found to decrease significantly ($P<0.01$) from the baseline area (7.2 ± 4.7 cm^2) to 4.4 ± 3.5 cm^2 after 8 weeks of therapy (Figure 17.3). About 10% of myomas did not appear to respond very well to GnRH analogue treatment; in this group, histological

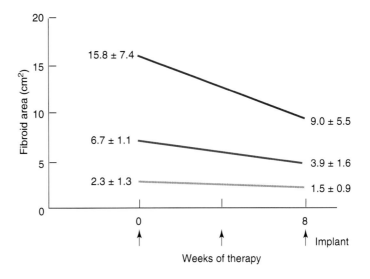

Figure 17.3 *Decrease in fibroid area after 8 weeks of GnRH agonist therapy relative to the initial value.*
——— *Myomas>10 cm^2*
——— *Myomas>5<10 cm^2*
═══ *Myomas<5 cm^2*

examination of the fibroids was required to exclude the rare occurrence of stromal endometrial tumours.

Operative techniques

The type of procedure depends on the type of submucous fibroid and the patient's desire to maintain childbearing capacities. When fertility is an issue, a myomectomy is performed electively; when the complaint is menorrhagia and fertility is no longer a consideration, an endometrial ablation may be performed with the myomectomy.

The maximum fibroid size for which a hysteroscopic procedure can be attempted is in the range of 7–8 cm. Beyond that size, depending on the patient's desire for maintaining fertility, the options of a myomectomy by minilaparotomy or laparoscopic subtotal hysterectomy are offered instead.

To facilitate cervical dilatation at the time of surgery, a 3–5 mm hygroscopic dilatator is inserted into the cervix the night before the operation. The patient is given the alternative of an epidural or general anaesthesia.

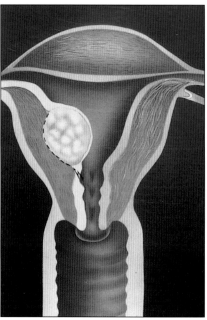

Figure 17.4 *Submucosal fibroids whose greatest diameter is inside the uterine cavity (reproduced with permission from Sutton & Diamond (eds)* Endoscopic Surgery for Gynaecologists, *W. B. Saunders & Co. Ltd, London, 1992).*

Submucous fibroids

Greatest diameter inside the uterine cavity (Figure 17.4)
In a series of 233 patients, the procedure was performed satisfactorily and, in straightforward conditions, only three cases presented particular difficulties. The myometrium overlying the fibroid was observed to be less vascular, and the shrinkage of the uterine cavity may have led to the relative ease with which the fibroids could be separated from the surrounding myometrium (Figure 17.5).

Removing the dissected fibroid from the cavity is not necessary: it can be left in the uterine cavity unless no decrease in size is observed after GnRH analogue therapy, in which case histological examination is mandatory. Leaving the fibroid *in situ* is not associated in our experience with infection, bleeding or uterine contractions. Presumably, the fibroid is expelled at the first menstruation after the discontinuation of GnRH agonist therapy. Indeed, an outpatient hysteroscopy performed 2–3 months after myomectomy has confirmed the complete disappearance of fibroids left in the cavity. When the fibroid is needed for histological examination, the cervix is further dilated with up to number 13–14 Hegar probes and the fibroid is simply extracted with ovum forceps. The fibroid can also be morcellated with the help of the laser fibre, the chips of fibroid being progressively removed until the cavity is cleared.

In our series, the operating time ranged from 10 to 50 min (mean 24 ± 6 min).

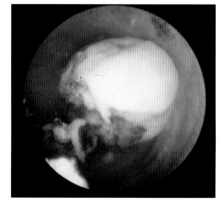

Figure 17.5 *Hysteroscopic view of the submucous fibroid, dissected off the myometrium with the fibre (reproduced with permission from Sutton & Diamond (eds)* Endoscopic Surgery for Gynaecologists, *W. B. Saunders & Co. Ltd, London, 1992).*

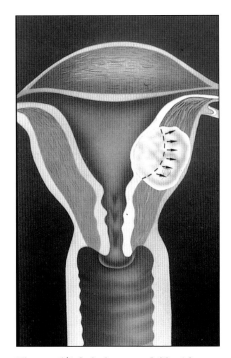

Figure 17.6 *Submucosal fibroids whose greatest diameter is inside the uterine wall (reproduced with permission from Sutton & Diamond (eds)* Endoscopic Surgery for Gynaecologists, *W. B. Saunders & Co. Ltd, London, 1992).*

Greatest diameter inside the uterine wall (Figure 17.6)

For large submucous fibroids whose greatest diameter is inside the uterine wall, a two-step operative hysteroscopy is proposed. After 8 weeks of preoperative GnRH analogue therapy, partial myomectomy is carried out through the hysteroscope by resecting the protruding portion of the fibroid. The laser fibre is then introduced into the intramural part of the remaining fibroid, to a depth of about 5–10 mm. During the application of laser energy, the fibre is slowly removed so that the deeper areas are coagulated. Endovaginal echography the day before surgery gives crucial information on fibroid size and the thickness of the uterine wall covering the external aspect of the intramural fibroid; being aware of this minimizes the risk of an unwanted perforation of the cavity. This firing procedure aims to reduce the size of the remaining fibroid by decreasing its vascularity and provoking an 'iatrogenic necrobiosis'[16]; this technique can be called transhysteroscopic myolysis.

After the first operative procedure, the patient is given another 8 week course of GnRH analogue therapy. At second-look operation, the hysteroscopic view of the cavity (Figure 17.7) shows a white avascular fibroid remnant protruding in the lumen, as if the shrinkage of the uterus induced by the continued GnRH analogue therapy had virtually expelled the residual necrotic fibroid; the laser fibre can then easily dissect off the remnant and complete the second step of the myomectomy. At the end of the procedure, the fibroid is again left in the uterine cavity. No concomitant laparoscopy is usually carried out,

Figure 17.7 *Second-look hysteroscopic view of an intramural fibroid, 8 weeks after transhysteroscopic myolysis; the intramural portion of the myoma protrudes inside the uterine cavity and will be easily dissected from the surrounding myometrium (reproduced with permission from Sutton & Diamond (eds)* Endoscopic Surgery for Gynaecologists, *W. B. Saunders & Co. Ltd, London, 1992).*

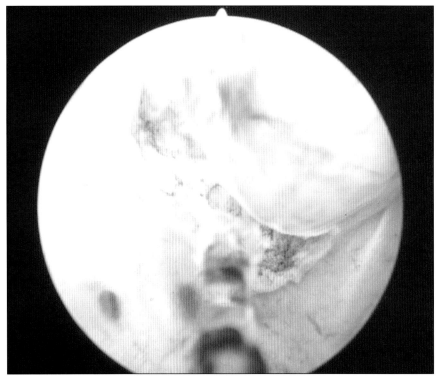

but it is an additional safeguard in certain cases. Microscopic examination of fibroids will reveal areas of necrosis.

Only in five cases was third-look hysteroscopy necessary to achieve a definitive myomectomy.

Hysterography and hysteroscopy typically reveal a normal appearance of the uterine cavity less than 3 months after the procedure.

Multiple fibroids

In multiple submucous fibroids, each is either separated from the surrounding myometrium or totally coagulated. When only a small portion is visible, the laser fibre is introduced into the intramural portion to a depth depending on the diameter of the fibroid (diagnosed by echography). While firing, the fibre is slowly removed. Each fibroid is systematically destroyed. At the end of surgery, endometrial ablation with the Nd-YAG laser is carried out to induce uterine shrinkage only in women older than 35 years who do not wish to become pregnant. In a multifibromatous uterus, the recurrence of menorrhagia associated with this technique has recently been estimated at 25%; therefore, when fertility preservation is no longer an issue in women over 40 years of age, laparoscopic subtotal hysterectomy can legitimately be proposed.

Operative results

Table 17.1 summarizes the long-term results according to the classification of Donnez and Nisolle[17]. Surgery was successful in 230 of 233 patients with large submucous fibroids whose greatest diameter was inside the uterine cavity. In three cases a stromal tumour was diagnosed. In one of these, dissection of the fibroid from the myometrium was impossible because the plane of dissection could not be found. Frozen-section histology of a biopsy revealed histological characteristics of stromal tumour, and vaginal hysterectomy was then carried out. The other two cases were diagnosed by histological examination of the removed fibroids, which appeared hysteroscopically benign. The incidence of stromal tumours in apparently benign fibroids is thus 1.3% (three of 233). All three tumours were observed in patients who did not respond very well (< 10% decrease) to GnRH analogue therapy.

Successful myomectomy permits the restoration of normal menstrual flow. Long-term results show that recurrence of menorrhagia occurs more frequently in patients with multiple submucous fibroids[15]. Recurrence of menorrhagia is provoked by the growth of fibroids on other sites, as shown by hysterography and hysteroscopy.

Our first evaluation[10] of 60 women with respect to subsequent fertility was published in 1990: 24 of the 60 treated women wished to

Table 17.1 *Surgical procedures and long-term results according to the site of myomas*

	Greatest diameter inside the uterine cavity	Largest portion located in the uterine wall	Multiple submucosal myomas (myomectomy and endometrial ablation)
Surgical procedures			
Total no. of patients	233	78	55
Successful	230	74	51
Failed	3*	4†	4‡
1 year follow-up			
Total no. of patients	132	42	39
Recurrence of menorrhagia	1 (1%)	1 (2%)	8 (20%)
2 year follow-up			
Total no. of patients	98	24	24
Recurrence of menorrhagia	2 (2%)	1 (4%)	6 (25%)

* Stromal tumor.
†Third-look hysteroscopy allowed the removal of the myoma.
‡Myomectomy was not totally successful. In two cases, second-look laser hysteroscopy was successfully performed. In the other two cases, vaginal hysterectomy was proposed and successfully performed).

become pregnant and had no other cause of infertility and, of the 24, 16 (67%) became pregnant within the first 8 months of recovery of menstruation. There were no miscarriages or preterm labour, and caesarean section was necessary because of fetal distress in one woman.

Discussion

The management of uterine fibroids remains surgical, as medical options have all failed to achieve definitive treatment. GnRH analogues have been documented to reduce uterine volume and fibroid volume on echography by 52–77% after 6 months of administration. Unfortunately, this reduction in size is often temporary and most leiomyomata return to pretreatment size within 4 months of cessation of therapy[18–21]. In our study, hysterographic evaluation of the uterine cavity size showed a reduction of 35% after 8 weeks of GnRH analogue administration[9,22]. A treatment duration of 8 weeks was adopted before hysteroscopic myomectomy, as the shrinkage of the uterine cavity area obtained after 8 weeks of therapy is not significantly different from that observed after 12 weeks of treatment. Another study[10] reported a mean reduction in fibroid volume of 38% (range 2–95%) following preoperative treatment by GnRH analogue for 8 weeks.

Besides the reduction in size of the fibroids, preoperative administration of GnRH analogues has several other advantages, as listed below. The risk of fluid overload is decreased. As endometrial vascularization may affect liquid resorption, the atrophic status of the endometrium induced by the GnRH agonists, together with a reduction in size of the cavity, will significantly limit the absorption of fluid. Reduction in myometrial vascularity as demonstrated by Doppler investigation of the uterine artery[23] also explains the minimal peroperative blood loss. By preventing uterine bleeding, preoperative GnRH analogue therapy permits the restoration of a normal haemoglobin concentration and makes later autologous transfusion a possibility. Failure to achieve any reduction in fibroid size or a poor response (less than 10% of the pretreatment size), a situation observed in nearly 10% of the patients in our series, draws attention to the possibility of a malignant condition; in such cases, extraction of the specimen for histological examination from the uterine cavity after myomectomy is mandatory. In our series, three stromal tumours were detected.

Advantages of preoperative GnRH administration

- Decreased risk of fluid overload
- Reduction in the size of fibroids
- Prevention of uterine bleeding
- Detection of a possible malignant condition if fibroid size is unaffected

---

The surgical technique is determined by the type of submucous fibroid, according to the hysterographic submucous classification of Donnez and Nisolle[12].

If the greatest diameter of the fibroid is inside the uterine cavity, hysteroscopic myomectomy is performed after an 8 week treatment with GnRH analogues. Unless no decrease in fibroid size is observed, the fibroid is left in the cavity; after a necrotic phase, the fibroid is probably expelled with menstrual blood.

When the greatest diameter of the fibroid is inside the uterine wall, myomectomy is carried out in two steps. Preoperative echography with an endovaginal transducer must be performed the day before surgery, to assess the distance between the deepest portion of the fibroid and the uterine serosa. With careful preoperative evaluation, there is no risk of damage to the bowel or the bladder by the transmural Nd-YAG energy effect. The pelvic structures are protected from injury because the distance between the tip of the fibre and the external surface of the uterus should never be less than 1.5 cm. There is no risk in inserting a laser fibre as much as 1 cm into the remaining portion if the diameter of the fibroid is more than 3–4 cm. During the first surgical stage, the protruding portion of the fibroid is removed and the intramural portion is devascularized by introducing the laser fibre into the fibroid, to a depth of 5–10 mm, depending on the depth of the remaining intramural portion. An additional GnRH analogue course is administered to allow the second stage to be performed 8 weeks later. A very interesting finding was that the intramural portion of the fibroid tends to become submucous and protrude into the uterine cavity. In all cases, at the second operation, the largest diameter of the remaining portion was inside the uterine cavity, so that a myomectomy was easily completed by separating it from the surrounding myometrium with the help of the Nd-YAG laser.

In the presence of multiple submucous fibroids, multiple myomectomy by hysteroscopy using the Nd-YAG laser after an 8 week course of GnRH therapy, has a higher recurrence rate in terms of menometrorrhagia, estimated in our series[15] at 25%; for this, laparoscopic subtotal hysterectomy is more suitable[24].

In conclusion, with the combined advantages of fibroid size reduction, the restoration of a normal haemoglobin level before operation, decreased risk of peroperative fluid overload and the detection of possible stromal tumours, GnRH analogue therapy is an effective adjunct to hysteroscopic surgery of submucous uterine fibroids.

Pretreatment hysteroscopy and directed endometrial biopsy help to rule out any neoplastic condition of the endomyometrium, which would contraindicate a conservative approach. In addition, hysterography on the day before surgery permits evaluation of the uterus and the fibroid size regression under the effect of the GnRH analogue; poor regression (less than 10% of the pretreatment size) suggests a stromal endometrial tumour and the fibroid specimen must then be sent for histology. In our series, even when the largest diameter of the myoma was in the myometrium, a two-step hysteroscopic procedure combined with GnRH agonist therapy represented the ideal management of large submucous fibroids[10,16], reducing the need for laparotomy, which is often accompanied by increased operative blood loss and postoperative adhesion formation[25].

Conclusion

Like Gallinat and Lueken[26], we believe that, although use of the Nd-YAG laser requires experience and a thorough knowledge of the technique, it nevertheless has a lower complication rate than use of the resectoscope. Nd-YAG laser treatment of large submucous fibroids must be considered the safest method for hysteroscopic surgical management of large fibroids.

Summary

Many patients with submucous fibroids can be safely treated by the hysteroscopic technique. Pre–operative diagnostic procedures including hysterography, outpatient hysteroscopy with directed endometrial biopsy and ultrasonography will identify those women with fibroids less than 8 cm in diameter and the relationship to the uterine cavity who are suitable for treatment. Pre–operative treatment with GnRH analogues will permit the reduction in size of the uterine cavity, size of the fibroid and the treatment of anaemia leading to faster, safer and more effective surgery. For larger fibroids, a two–stage treatment is advised, the second operation being performed eight weeks later. Recurrence of menorrhagia is more likely to occur if there have been multiple fibroids. Nd–YAG laser treatment is considered to be safer than the use of the resectoscope

References

1. MacLucas B (1991) Intrauterine applications of the resectoscope. *Surg Gynecol Obstet* **172**: 425.
2. Serden SP, Brooks PG (1991) Treatment of abnormal uterine bleeding with the gynaecological resectoscope. *J Reprod Med* **36**: 697.
3. Ke RW, Taylor PJ (1991) Endometrial ablation to control excessive uterine bleeding. *Hum Reprod* **6**: 574.
4. Baggish MS (1988) New laser hysteroscope for neodymium-YAG endometrial ablation. *Lasers Surg Med* **8**: 99.
5. Loffer FD (1988) Laser ablation of the endometrium. *Obstet Gynecol Clin North Am* **15**: 77.
6. Jacques SL (1992) Laser–tissue interactions: photochemical, photothermal and photomechanical. *Surg Clin North Am* **72**: 531.
7. Goldrath MH, Fuller T, Segal S (1981) Laser photovaporization of endometrium for the treatment of menorrhagia. *Am J Obstet Gynecol* **140**: 14.
8. Goldrath MH (1985). Hysteroscopic laser surgery. In: Baggish MG (ed.) *Basic and Advanced Laser Surgery in Gynaecology*. Appleton-Century-Crofts, Norwalk, p. 357.
9. Donnez J, Schrurs B, Gillerot S, Sadow J, Clerckx F (1989) Treatment of uterine fibroids with implants of gonadotrophin-releasing hormone agonist: assessment by hysterography. *Fertil Steril* **51**: 947.
10. Donnez J, Gillerot S, Bourgonjon D, Clerckx F, Nisolle M (1990) Neodymium:YAG laser hysteroscopy in large submucous fibroids. *Fertil Steril* **54**: 999.

11. Nisolle M, Grandjean P, Gillerot S, Donnez J (1991) Endometrium ablation with the Nd:YAG laser in dysfunctional bleeding. *Minimal Invasive Therapy* **1**: 35.

12. Donnez J, Nisolle M (1994) Hysteroscopic lysis of intrauterine adhesions (Asherman's syndrome). In: Donnez J, Nisolle M (eds) *An Atlas of Laser Operative Laparoscopy and Hysteroscopy*. Parthenon Publishing, London, p. 305.

13. Nisolle M, Donnez J (1994) Mullerian fusion defects: septoplasty and hemihysterectomy of the rudimentary horns. In: Donnez J, Nisolle M (eds) *An Atlas of Laser Operative Laparoscopy and Hysteroscopy*. Parthenon Publishing, London, p. 295.

14. Neuwirth RS (1983) Hysteroscopic management of symptomatic submucous fibroids. *Obstet Gynecol* **62**: 509.

15. Donnez J (1993) Nd:YAG laser hysteroscopic myomectomy. In: Sutton C, Diamond M (eds) *Endoscopic Surgery for Gynaecologists*. W.B. Saunders, London, p. 331.

16. Donnez J, Nisolle M (1992) Hysteroscopic surgery. *Curr Opin Obstet Gynecol* **4**: 439.

17. Donnez J, Nisolle M (1993) Nd-YAG laser hysteroscopic surgery: endometrial ablation, partial endometrial ablation and myomectomy. *Reprod Med Rev* **2**: 63.

18. Healy DL, Fraser HM, Lawson SL (1984) Shrinkage of a uterine fibroid after subcutaneous infusion of a LHRH agonist. *Br Med J* **209**: 267.

19. Maheux R, Guilloteau C, Lemay A, Bastide A, Fazekas ATA (1985) Luteinizing hormone-releasing hormone agonist and uterine leiomyoma: pilot study. *Am J Obstet Gynecol* **152**: 1034.

20. Andreyko JL, Blumenfeld Z, Marschall LA, Monroe SE, Hricak H, Jaffe RB (1988) Use of an agonistic analogue of gonadotrophin-releasing hormone (nNafarelin) to treat leiomyomas: assessment by magnetic resonance imaging. *Am J Obstet Gynecol* **158**: 903.

21. Friedman AJ, Barbieri RL, Doubilet PM, Fine C, Schiff I (1988) A randomized, double-blind trial of gonadotrophin releasing-hormone agonist (leuprolide) with or without medroxyprogesterone acetate in the treatment of leiomyomata uteri. *Fertil Steril* **49**: 404.

22. Donnez J, Clerckx F, Gillerot S, Bourgonjon D, Nisolle M (1989) Traitement des fibromes uterins par implant d'agoniste de la GnRH: evaluation par hysterographie. *Contrac Fertil Sex* **17**: 569.

23. Matta WHM, Stabile I, Shaw RS, Campbell S (1988) Doppler assessment of uterine blood flow changes in patients with fibroids receiving the gonadotrophin-releasing hormone agonist buserelin. *Fertil Steril* **49**: 1083.

24. Donnez J, Nisolle M (1993) Laparoscopic supracervical (subtotal) hysterectomy (LASH). *J Gynaecol Surg* **9**: 91–4.

25. Berkeley AS, DeCherney AH, Polan ML (1983) Abdominal myomectomy and subsequent fertility. *Surg Gynecol Obstet* **156**: 319.

26. Gallinat A (1993) Hysteroscopic treatment of submucous fibroids using the Nd:YAG laser and modern electrical equipment. In: Leuken RP, Gallinat A (eds) *Endoscopic Surgery in Gynaecology*. Demeter Verlag, Berlin, pp. 72–8.

Index